CELL, GENE AND MOLECULAR THERAPY: NEW CONCEPTS

CELL, GENE AND MOLECULAR THERAPY: NEW CONCEPTS

VIROJ WIWANITKIT

Nova Biomedical Books
New York

For permission to use material from this book please contact us:
Telephone 631-231-7269; Fax 631-231-8175
Web Site: http://www.novapublishers.com

LIBRARY OF CONGRESS CATALOGING-IN-PUBLICATION DATA

Viroj Wiwanitkit.
Cell, gene, and molecular therapy : new concepts / Viroj Wiwanitkit.
p. ; cm.
Includes bibliographical references and index.
ISBN 978-1-60692-532-4 (hardcover)
1. Therapeutics, Experimental. 2. Cellular therapy. 3. Immunotherapy. 4. Gene therapy. I. Title.
[DNLM: 1. Therapeutics. WB 300 V821c 2009]
RM111.V57 2009
615.8'95--dc22

2008047192

Published by Nova Science Publishers, Inc. ✦ New York

CONTENTS

PREFACE

Treatment is the heart of medicine. For patient, the main aim of visiting to the physician is to get the best therapy. Therapy has a long history. At the present, advanced biotechnology help improve the medical treatment. Apart from the classical treatment, there are many new emerging means of medical treatment. In this book, the concept of new therapeutic channels, cell, gene and molecular concepts will be focused. Interesting details on concepts for these modern therapies can be found in this book and this book can be the reference resource for the physician, medical personnel and health care worker for update the knowledge of treatment.

Chapter I - Health is the best wealth. Everyone requires good health to maintain his/her daily life. In general, everyone will be healthy if there is no external or internal insult to disturb his/her normal physiological function. There are several possible insults that can bring problem to one's health. The insult can be biological, chemical or physical. Examples of biological insults are pathogen, germ, parasite, organic substances and etc. Examples of chemical insults are chemical substances and toxins. Examples of physical insults are electrical power, mechanical power, radioactive power and etc.

For developing an overt abnormality, there will be a classical process. Molecular or submolecular changes will accumulate to form a biochemical change. Biochemical changes will accumulate to form a physiological change. Physiological changes will accumulate to form an anatomical change. Anatomical changes will accumulate to form overt abnormality. This step by step process is the core concept in medicine. This concept is also applicable to the concept of advanced bioinformatics. To study on a disease, probing to a wide range on its pathogenesis can be done by modern bioinformatics concept. From gene to protein to expression can be manipulated. Geneomics makes use of genome data to explain genomic phenomenon. Proteomics makes uses of proteome data to explain proteomic phenomenon. There are also other "omics" sciences that can be used. The other omics sciences are transcriptomics, metabolomics, cytomics and etc. If readers feel interested on these new omics sciences, suggestion is made for reading textbook on bioinformatics science.

Focusing on the work "disease", it covers a wide range of disorders. Disease is usually used for describing any overt abnormalities. Disease usually means any conditions that need proper medical management or treatment. It should be noted that some abnormalities, especially for those in molecular level change, will not be called disease. Healthy in general means no disease. However, as previously mentioned, molecular level abnormalities can be existed and this brings the stage of pre-disease or risk. The current concept in medicine moves to prevention rather than treatment. In preventive medicine, finding for risk is necessary and proper management on identified risk must be done.

The study of the relation of man to his/her environment in developing countries emphasizes the inevitable need for societies to know the true causes of infection, malnutrition, and poverty. The requirement is for improvement in the quality of human life in less developed nations, a recommendation easy to prescribe but hard to accomplish. The present focus includes the relation between economic and other factors in health development. This interpretation has been selected for the acceptance of a disciplinary approach in the commissioning of papers might have the unintended effect of excluding some key areas of study, which makes use of the consideration of crucial interrelationships between disciplines. Nutrition as a discipline evolved out of medical and bio-chemical concept on the relation between food and health. Until the 1950s nutrient deficiencies dominated the nutritional track of analysis. From this moment attention was further led to nutritional consequences of the welfare state. The interrelation between health, nutrition and welfare is complex.

Chapter II - Nanotechnology is a modern technology covering to management, construction, synthesis of devices in atomic or molecular level that has its the size between, 1 and 100 nanometers. The nanodevice has its special function in physical, chemical and biological aspect that can be adapted for usage. Nanotechnology is the application of knowledge on nanoscience. Nanoscience is a modern science covering on the natural fact of nanolevel conditions. Nanoscience focuses on three main scientific areas: physical, chemical and biological sciences. The main fundamental knowledge for the beginner in nanoscience is what nanolevel is. "Nano" is a modern scientific work describing for the 10^{-9} level. The nanolevel is minuteder or fewer than microlevel (micro = 10^{-6}). Nanotechnologies can assist practitioner diagnosis at the single-cell and molecule levels, and some can be adapted in current molecular diagnostic methods, such as biochips. Nanoparticles, such as gold nanoparticles, silver nanoparticles and quantum dots, are the most broadly used, but various other nanotechnological devices for manipulation at the nanoscale as well as nanobiosensors are also promising for potential clinical applications. In conclusion, nanotechnologies will expand the borders of current molecular diagnostics and assist in point-of-care diagnostics, integration of diagnostics with therapeutics, and modern construction of personalized medicine. Jain mentioned for the emerging role of advances in biochip and microarray technologies in the modern construction of personalized medicine. Jain proposed that biochips such as GeneChip, CYP450, electrochemical biochips, protein biochips, microfluidic biochips and nanotechnology-based biochips played a significant role in molecular diagnostics, and their application in point-of-care diagnosis is expected to facilitate the modern construction of personalized medicine. Although the potential diagnostic applications are wildly expanded, the most important current applications are limited in the areas of biomarker discomuch, cancer diagnosis, and determination of infectious pathogens.

Chapter III - Quantum is a physical term that implies the smallest discrete amount of some physical property that a system can have. Quantum theory, the branch of physics which is based on quantization, started in 1900 when Planck published his theory explaining the emission spectrum of black bodies. The bippoasesic of radiation as well as matter is the heart of the quantum theory. In physics, quantum mechanics is the learning of the relationship between energy or radiation as well as matter, in particular that between valence shell electrons as well as photons. Bohr's theory is the root for the generation of the present quantum physics. Bohr's atomic theory is broadly viewed as remarkable, both for its accuracy in predicting the observed optical transitions of one-electron atoms as well as for its failure to fully correspond with current electronic structure theory. However, what is not routinely appreciated is that Bohr's classical semiclassical conception differed significantly from the Bohr-Sommerfeld theory as well as offers an alternative semiclassical approximation scheme with remarkable attributes. It is routinely believed that the old quantum theory, as presented by Bohr in 1913, fails when adapted to few electron systems, such as the H(2) molecule. Bohr's classical method did not impose action quantization constraints but rather obtained these as predictions by simply matching photon as well as classical orbital frequencies. The discovery of the efficacy-quantum by Planck as well as further work of Borh was the fundamental contributing root to Einstein's hypothesis of lightquanta. With the mentioned fundamental theories, Einstein could explain the external light-electrical effect. The work of Einstein is the root of the modern ppoasese of science. As a case study, there was a long track from the concept of stimulated emission as the fundamental idea of laser technical work by Albert Einstein in 1917 to the practical use of the laser are present. It is also the fundamental for the modern science, quantum mechanics. Quantum mechanics is a fundamental branch of physics with wide applications in both experimental as well as theoretical physics. The quantum theory is the theoretical basis of modern physics that can be valuable in explaining the nature as well as behavior of matter as well as energy on the atomic as well as subatomic level. Conrad said that biological cells had greater information processing efficiency than the programmable computers used to model them. Conrad also suggested that systems in which quantum features played a prominent work are more powerful than classical physical-dynamical analogs.

Quantum medicine is the modern kind of medicine. Naturally, all things, chemicals, plants, animals as well as human beings are composed of various tissues, organs, cells, molecules, as well as atoms. The combinations of atoms lead to molecules. The combinations of molecules lead to cells. The combinations of cells results in tissues. The combinations of tissues lead to organs. The combinations of organs lead to human beings. Fundamentally, an atom consists of electron as well as nuclei which intern quantum as well as neutron. Electron poses negative charge, proton poses positive charge as well as neutron poses neutral charge. Normally human beings cannot see the atom. In addition, the compositions of atom are beyond human reach. But according to the modern elementary particle theory, elementary particle is considered to have immense size as well as types, as well as it poases property as energy field which rotates as well as vibrates itself. With the advent in nanoscience, those very tiny compositions can be studied.

Quantum determination method is the determination technique, which tests the energy composed of magnetic energy generated by quantum as well as electron movement. Improvements in quantum chemical techniques have led to increased applications to biological problems, including the generation of potential energy functions for molecular mechanics as well as modeling of the reactive chemistry in enzyme active sites, with particularly interesting progress being constructed for metal-containing systems. The three items to be considered in quantum determination method are (a) use of quantum mechanical electronic structure techniques such as molecular orbital theory as well as density functional theory, usually in conjunction with molecular mechanics; (b) treating vibrational motions quantum mechanically, either in an instantaneous harmonic approximation, or by path integrals, or by a three-dimensional wave function coupled to classical nuclear motion; (c) incorporation of multidimensional tunneling approximations into reaction rate calculations. Orbital theory is the fundamental knowledge for quantum chemistry. Molecular orbital analytical work is the fundamental technique for study of quantum mechanical electronic structure. To assist molecular orbital analytical work, there are several modern computation instruments for performing this analytical aim. As a case study, AOMix is a modern user-friendly software for the molecular orbital analytical work. It calculates the molecular orbital compositions in terms of the constituent chemical parts in the molecule or atom. AOMix automatically processes output files of multiple quantum-chemical packages. AOMix also permits to deeply review chemical structure making use of overlap populations (total as well as per molecular orbital), valence indices, 2-center (Mayer, Lowdin, Wiberg, as well as bond-order symmetry components) as well as 3- as well as 4-center bond orders, charge decomposition orbital, CDA (total, per molecular orbital, per symmetry type), as well as condensed Fukui functions. Conventional quantum chemistry techniques are either too expensive to apply to large systems or too approximate for the results to be reliable, as well as they fail to satisfy this requirement. A variety of different approaches is being developed with the aim of achieving this goal: local correlation techniques; divide-as well as-conquer techniques; linear-scaling density functional techniques based on the fast multiple as well as other approximations; effective potential techniques; as well as hybrid techniques.

The influence as well as application of quantum determination on medical field is named "quantum medicine". Quantum medicine is one of the most promising tracks of modern contemporary medicine. It is based on the use of aimful effects of low-dosage electromagnetic radiation or quantum in treatment, diagnosis, prophylaxis, as well as rehabilitation of patients.

Chapter IV – Engineering is a specific science that focuses mainly on the physical aspect. There are man fields of engineering at present. For example, electrical engineering is a specific branch of engineering dealing with electricity. However, due to the concept of convergence of science, engineering becomes emerged with biological science. Application of engineering in biological science helps jump across the inter-science barrier and brings new advent to the world population. For example, merging between computational engineering and genetics biology brings new science called genomics [1-3], which is the modern blooming science at present. Nanoengineering plus medicine forms nanomedicine which is another present new hope of the world for global health development.

Application of engineering on biology helps explain and manipulate difficult biological question. This can be applied in medicine, which is a branch of biological science. Special forms of medical applications can be seen. One of the most famous application is medical engineering. This involves medical instrumentation as well as other applied engineering for medicine. As mentioned, the usefulness of application of engineering in medicine is very much. It helps from diagnosis, treatment and prevention. In this book, the author focuses content on treatment, therefore, treatment will be focused and applied engineering for treatment in medicine will be mentioned. An important therapeutic application is tissue engineering and medical biopolymer science. The application is useful for reconstructive medicine. Specifically, medical biopolymers are presently used in dentistry and orthopedics. With these applications, it can help manage previously untreatable diseases and conditions. Further details will be further discussed.

Chapter V - When an organ lost, it is necessary to get medical management. Organ lost usually means lost of function. In severe case, organ lost ends up with death. There is no method to recover in the past and this has been continuously searched for the solution. Transplantation is a new concept using the replacement of the lost organs by the new ones. New ones means new organ from the others. Therefore, it means transferring of one's organ to another. This is ethical concern and new concept in medicine. Indeed, organ transplantation has long history. More than 50 years are recorded. Learning of history of transplantation is necessary to allow us to appreciate the great potential offered by current biomedical science and engineering for future developments in the therapies of this more than natural practice. At present, embryonic stem cells are used in the studies of the differentiation of various cells or tissues for transplantation therapy, because of their pluripotential property to differentiate into almost all types of cells in the body.

Chapter VI - Radioactive substance is classified as a new group of elements that human beings knew for about 1 century. After the discovery of Curie Family, radioactive substance becomes on focused interested of global scientist. There are many researches on radioactive substance. Application of radioactive substance for usage is continuously proposed. At present, radioactive substances can be used in industry as well as medicine. The main focus of radioactive use in medicine is for treatment of tumor. Also it is applied for diagnosis as radioassay.

Parallel to radioactive substance, rays are also focused for its application in medicine. After the discovery of X-ray, the application in medicine is a big jump of medical world. With use of X-ray, physician can visualize the internal structure of human being and used it for diagnosis. This is the history of development of a famous medical science, radiology. At present, radiology is a necessary medical science that helps both diagnose and treat of patients. Radiology unit is a basic unit for all hospital. Basically, three basic main branches of radiology are described as radiodiagnosis, radiotherapy and nuclear medicine. Radiodiagnosis focuses mainly on diagnosis of disorders by usage of several means of imaging technology in medicine. Radiotherapy focuses mainly on treatment and will be mainly detailed and discussed in this chapter. Finally, nuclear medicine focuses mainly on both diagnosis and treatment based on usage of radioactive substances. Important details of nuclear medicine based treatment will also be detailed and discussed in this chapter.

Chapter VII - "God made the sun. God made the moon. God made the star." These sentences are basic principle for Christian. Living things in the worlds started for many million years ago. Nobody can tell the exact starting point of time for life. Life is complex. Generation of living thing is a very complicated process and no present high technology can work this. Natural makes life. This can be said that god made life. Due to Buddhism, life can be generated if there are fulfill criteria. as a) father and mother have sexual intercourse, b) the time is proper and c) there must be specific superstitious spirit for this condition. This is the fact. There must be gametes from both mother and father for fertilization. In human, beginning of new lie is widely studied. After fertilization, development process in utero is continuous. Embryonic generation is a developmental process for all human beings. Everyone in this world had to pass this step before birth. Further process as passing from embryo to fetus is the next step in utero. Birth is the finalized process for in utero processes and this is the starting point of human status.

Considering the embryonic period, the generation of cell and tissue is the main hallmark activity. Of several processes, first sign of life, movement, can be seen at the third month after fertilization. For cell and tissue growth, basic promoter as stem cell is required. Stem cell is the basic cell generator of other cells and tissues. This is also the important step in development for starting of complete life. Stem cell has its main function during in utero period. However, some stem cell is still existed and functional in full term human life. This can be seen in bone marrow, which is the source of generation of blood cell in circulation. It is accepted that blood cell must be generated all times thorough the life of human beings. Harvesting stem cell for medical use is the present focus. It can be important and applied for treatment process of some previously untreatable diseases. Stem cell technology could also be a significant helpful tool for an understanding on early human developmental process and screening potential candidates for new drug search.

Chapter VIII - There are many basic case groups to receive extensive blood transfusions including the cases in intensive care unit, thalassemic cases, acute blood lost cases as well as traumatic cases. Approximately four-fifth get multiple transfusions. At present donor exposure is an issue because transfusion risk is still apparent. Gived blood should be applied for the treatment of cases as well as poses well asled with the same serious respect as well as ethical stas well asards as with which it was gived by the donor. Directed donor or purcposesed system should not be encouraged. Anonymous donation should be applied. As a rule blood msut be given as a gift with no reimbursement as well as should be applied to an unknown case with the intention to help as well as not to harm. Donation shall be easy as well as secure for the donor. Therefore, blood shall be poses well asled with respect as well as should be applied with the intension to treat cases as previouly stated. Promotion of the blood donation is the topic. Owing to a recent study, the principal obstacle for blood donation is fear owing to poor knowledge.

Gived blood have to be applied for treatment of case directly or indirectly. Direct help to the case might be transfusion of single units or transfusion of units from a batch, platelets or plasma outcomes. Indirect help to the case include using of a few tubes for laboratory controls or many units for stas well asards with the intention to help cases to set normal values for a new test which is useful for laboratory medicine. Use of gived blood for other aims than transfusion have to be no specific information when blood is applied as laboratory quality controls but information for other kinds of use as well as assure for no identification at the pposese of informed consent with identification of donor is needed.

Chapter IX - Light is a basic thing that human beings know. Light is mainly from the sun. Electricity can also provide light. Therapy by light is also a medical concept. Since light poses energy therefore it might be used for treatment. In this chapter, the author will present the topic on phototherapy. Main kinds of application, photodynamic therapy and classical phototherapy for newborn will be discussed.

Chapter X - At the starting point of this century genetics arose out of developmental history as the science of the reasonable understanding of development. The concept of the difference between the possibility for a trait and the trait proper, between the genotype and the phenotype, was clear only during the first decade of the century. After Spemann's epochal discovery, who already rewarded with the Nobel Prize in 1935, of the organizer and the beginning of the experimental analysis of developmental fields, little or no progress was derived until the last few years when a new emerging revolution appeared in developmental biology. The classical point of view prevailed into the 1930s, and conceived the gene as an indivisible single item of genetic transmission, recombination, mutation, and function. The discovery of intragenic recombination in the early 1940s and the setting of DNA as the physical basis of inheritance resulted in the neoclassical concept of the gene, which prevailed until the 1970s.

In the past, studying of the gene is not easy but very difficult. Genetic laboratory seems to be a complex and mysterious field. The discoveries of DNA technology, beginning in the early 1970s, have resulted in the second revolution in the concept of the gene in which none of the classical or neoclassical criteria for the definition of the gene hold extremely true. These are several new findings concerning gene repetition and overlapping, movable genes, complex promoters, multiple polyadenylation sites, polyprotein genes, editing of the primary transcript, pseudogenes and gene nesting. Introduction of Southern, Northern and dot blotting and DNA sequencing later in the 1970s considerably improved the diagnostic capabilities. Nevertheless, it was the new finding of the polymerase chain reaction (PCR) in 1985 that resulted in an exponential blooming in molecular biology and the introduction of practicable nucleic acid tests in the routine laboratory. Blooming of molecular biology leads to several simplified techniques for genetic studying. Finding amino acid sequence of a gene can be easily done by basic sequencing technique.

Chapter XI – The word immunity is a basic medical word describing a specific system of human beings. Immunity is a specific system dealing with the defensive mechanism. Everyday, human body has to expose to several alien foreign bodies and some of these alien foreign bodies are harmful and needs proper management. Immunity plays important roles for this overall process. Considering defensive mechanism of human beings, there are 2 main parts immunity and non-immunity portions. Non-immunity portion is a non specific process and usually firstly act to any alien foreign bodies. Examples of non specific process are mucous barrier and several reflexes. Considering immunity, it is a specific process. The hallmarks of immunity consists of memory and specificity, therefore, the first exposure cannot generate immunity. The immunity process can be divided into two main parts: humoral mediated immunity and cellular mediated immunity. Humoral medicated immunity makes use of humoral substance, antibody for action. Whereas cellular mediated immunity makes use of cells, blood cells, for action. Of several cells in blood stream, lymphocyte, T cell, B cell and nonTnonB cell, are mentioned for cellular mediated immunity. These main kinds of lymphocytes take important role in cellular immune process. T cell takes role for generation of cytokine whereas B cell takes roles in antibody generation process.

As mentioned, immunity plays main roles in defensive mechanism. When a foreign body enters into human body and pass non specific immune defensive mechanism process, it will be further reacted by immunity. Destruction of foreign body can be seen via antibody system with help of compliment or via cell mediated immunity process with help of cytokine. With complete full function of immunity, pathogens or foreign bodies can be successfully destroyed. However, in some cases, those aliens can conquer immune system process and this will result in pathological conditions or diseases. Good examples are infections. With complete perfect immunity, human will be helpful. However, extremely high immunity process or hypersensitivity can be problematic. On the other hand, extremely low immunity process of immunity or immunodeficiency can also be problematic.

Chapter XII – Vaccine is a specific important tool in medicine. Due to the principle of immunity, human beings require immune to defend any alien foreign bodies. However, immunity cannot be functional if there is no previous exposure. This means it has to be a memory before immune generation or the human beings must experience previous foreign bodies' invasion. However, in some cases, immunity is slightly generated and cannot fight with external invasion of align foreign bodies and this brings mortality and morbidity. Therefore, simulating the invasion of align foreign bodies to prepare for real invasion is needed and very useful. This is the concept of vaccination. Vaccination is defined as a primary prevention. Vaccine can prevent before real existence. Vaccine is a mode of simulating interaction as previously described.

Vaccination is classified as an active immunization. This means tit makes uses of human beings physiological process to create immune by itself. There are several vaccine at present. Recommendation for vaccination might be different in different settings. Expanded Program on Immunization (EPI) is the basic public health one in all countries. With use of vaccine, controls of many infectious diseases are feasible. Pox is an example of infectious disease that can be controlled by vaccine. This infection is already got rid of by succeed in global vaccination. The presently widely used vaccine include rabies vaccine, measles vaccine, rubella vaccine, Japanese encephalitis vaccine, hepatitis B vaccine, hepatitis A vaccine, influenza vaccine, varicella vaccine, pneumococcal vaccine, pertussis vaccine, diphtheria vaccine, BCG and toxiod. However, at present, there are attempts to develop more vaccines for real clinical usage/. This is the aim of preventive medicine. In addition, there are attempts to develop vaccine for expanded usefulness. This is the origin of therapeutic vaccine. This is the new trend to use vaccine as treatment tool. This is classified as immunotherapy. The details of this new way of immunotherapy will be further detailed and discussed in this chapter. To produce a therapeutic vaccine, it might be a basic knowledge on biotechnology and immunology. More details on this item can be seen in this chapter.

Chapter XIII - Terminology, chaperone means an adult who takes care of one or more unmarried men or women during social occasions. But this is not the medical specific meaning. In medicine, chaperone therapy is a new concept. Helping or assisting on other molecules is also the ways that chaperone acts. This term is primarily used in molecular biology. "How do chaperones operate in cells?" is a big scientific question. Saibil said that recent advances were giving an improved understanding of the nature of chaperone interactions with their non-native substrate proteins.

Burston and Clarke said that chaperones could be broadly defined as proteins which interact with non-native states of other protein molecules and this activity was significant in the folding of newly synthesized polypeptides and the assembly of multisubunit structures; the maintenance of proteins in unfolded states fit for translocation across membranes; and the stabilization of inactive appearances of proteins which are switched on by cellular signals; and the stabilization of proteins unfolded during cellular stress. Hartl said that different types of molecular chaperones, such as the members of the Hsp70 and Hsp60 families of heat-shock proteins, participate in a coordinated pathway of cellular protein folding.

Basically, Hsp70 proteins are central components of the cellular network of molecular chaperones and folding catalysts and these proteins could help a large variety of protein folding actions in the cell by transient relation to their substrate binding domain with short hydrophobic peptide segments within their substrate proteins. Hsp90 is another molecular chaperone related to the folding of signal-transducing proteins, such as steroid hormone receptors and protein kinases. Hsp90 contributes to several discrete subcomplexes, each having distinct groups of co-chaperones that function in folding pathways. Wegele et al. said that the chaperones Hsp70 and Hsp90 might have a function in the folding and maturation of key regulatory proteins, like steroid hormone receptors, transcription factors, and kinases, some of which were related to cancer progression. They noted that Hsp70 and Hsp90 construct a multichaperone complex, in which both are jointed by a third protein called Hop and such connection of and the interplay between the two chaperone machineries was of significant importance for cell viability. Callebaut et al. noted that domain III, common to the hsp60s and hsp70s was also found in the hsp90s and adopts a beta-alpha-beta Rossmann-folded structure which was enrolled in the NAD-binding domain of dehydrogenases. They noted that the hsp molecules could act as unfoldases by disrupting secondary structures through redox reactions on the main polypeptidic chain with which these molecules interact.

Chapter I

BASIC PRINCIPLE OF MEDICAL TREATMENT

HEALTHY AND DISEASE

A. General Concept

Health is the best wealth. Everyone requires good health to maintain his/her daily life. In general, everyone will be healthy if there is no external or internal insult to disturb his/her normal physiological function. There are several possible insults that can bring problem to one's health. The insult can be biological, chemical or physical. Examples of biological insults are pathogen, germ, parasite, organic substances and etc. Examples of chemical insults are chemical substances and toxins. Examples of physical insults are electrical power, mechanical power, radioactive power and etc.

For developing an overt abnormality, there will be a classical process. Molecular or submolecular changes will accumulate to form a biochemical change. Biochemical changes will accumulate to form a physiological change. Physiological changes will accumulate to form an anatomical change. Anatomical changes will accumulate to form overt abnormality. This step by step process is the core concept in medicine. This concept is also applicable to the concept of advanced bioinformatics. To study on a disease, probing to a wide range on its pathogenesis can be done by modern bioinformatics concept. From gene to protein to expression can be manipulated. Geneomics makes use of genome data to explain genomic phenomenon. Proteomics makes uses of proteome data to explain proteomic phenomenon. There are also other "omics" sciences that can be used. The other omics sciences are transcriptomics, metabolomics, cytomics and etc. If readers feel interested on these new omics sciences, suggestion is made for reading textbook on bioinformatics science.

Focusing on the work "disease", it covers a wide range of disorders. Disease is usually used for describing any overt abnormalities. Disease usually means any conditions that need proper medical management or treatment. It should be noted that some abnormalities, especially for those in molecular level change, will not be called disease. Healthy in general means no disease. However, as previously mentioned, molecular level abnormalities can be existed and this brings the stage of pre-disease or risk. The current concept in medicine moves to prevention rather than treatment. In preventive medicine, finding for risk is necessary and proper management on identified risk must be done.

The study of the relation of man to his/her environment in developing countries emphasizes the inevitable need for societies to know the true causes of infection, malnutrition, and poverty [1]. The requirement is for improvement in the quality of human life in less developed nations, a recommendation easy to prescribe but hard to accomplish [1]. The present focus includes the relation between economic and other factors in health development [2]. This interpretation has been selected for the acceptance of a disciplinary approach in the commissioning of papers might have the unintended effect of excluding some key areas of study, which makes use of the consideration of crucial interrelationships between disciplines [2]. Nutrition as a discipline evolved out of medical and bio-chemical concept on the relation between food and health [3]. Until the 1950s nutrient deficiencies dominated the nutritional track of analysis [3]. From this moment attention was further led to nutritional consequences of the welfare state [3]. The interrelation between health, nutrition and welfare is complex.

B. Health and Nutrition

It is accepted that nutritional status can reflex health status. In the 1980s, communication between anthropology and demography has increased broadly [4]. Methodological advances in demography have helped anthropologists conquer problematic aspects in describing and estimating parameters of populations [4]. New techniques include determinations of demographic parameters from the close study of kinship, computer simulations, model life tables, and other techniques in paleodemography [4]. Early malnutrition has been broadly associated with chronic diseases later in life [5]. The finding of metabolic disorders in individuals with malnutrition in fetal life and early in postnatal life may have significant public health implications in developing countries, although only a few researches have examined the relationship between body weight at the first year of life and later metabolic abnormalities [5]. At this moment it is necessary to proactively discuss and promote healthy eating behaviors among children at an early age and reassure parents to promote children's ability to self-regulate energy ingestion while providing proper structure and boundaries around eating [6]. The changes that are existent in body composition during ageing are described and how this may affect reduce risk [7]. The possible metabolic processes behind weight loss are discussed and many other factors that affect nutritional status in the older age group are described [7]. A life-course approach to chronic-disease epidemiology can make use of a multidisciplinary framework to understand the importance of time and timing in associations between exposures and results at the individual and population levels [8]. Due to this approach, health and nutrition has a very strong correlation [9]. "Does public health strategy give consideration to the manner of nutrition and its consequences for health?" is the main present question [9].

C. Health and Welfare

Heath and welfare has a closed correlation. The association between morbidity and mortality indicators and low socio-economic status has been observed for many centuries [10]. Although the 1979 report of the Royal Commission on the National Health Service upheld the public organization of a free health service in Britain, it did not bring a comprehensive retrospective view of the relationship between health experience, health goals, and health service policies [11]. Changes of life style resulting from rapid economic growth are suspected to be significant causes of the change in the prevalence of tuberculosis and acute gastrointestinal infectious disorders [12]. As for medical care services, several new medical requirements have emerged in recent years, including "quality of life," "palliative medicine in terminal care," "establishment of a primary care system" and "comprehensive care connecting health and medical care with welfare" etc [12]. Improved living standards resulting from economic growth, called the "economic miracle" internationally, have assisted to bring about a rapid and wide range of change in daily lifestyle, such as ingestion habits, working conditions and environment [12]. Hill said that the destruction of health infrastructure resulted in a loss of structures and processes that would otherwise protect prospective research subjects who are part of vulnerable populations [13]. More and more attention in several areas of medical activities is being used to the social aspects, for both individual and society levels, of these activities, and there is a drift from applied sociology towards medical one [14]. In spite of the cessations of the development of medical sociology as separate branch of sciences, the researches of recent years are demonstrating obvious approaching modern study issues and means, which do exist in contemporary world [14]. It identifies the growth of health systems research as part of a trend towards sectoral and programmatic development assistance, the emergence of new knowledge generation as a form of research linked to development, and the feasibility for conflict where multilateral and bilateral donors are both primary funders and users of health systems report [13].

D. Nutrition and Welfare

Nutrition can be the result of welfare management. The effect is well demonstrated in the pediatric population. Chaudhuri said that young children spend more than 90% of their time in the household environment, a specific place of exposure to hazardous substances [15]. Chaudhuri also said that childhood diarrheal disease and acute lower respiratory infections in the developing world represented a large portion of the global burden of disease and are strongly related to housing conditions [15]. In addition, Chaudhuri mentioned that allergies and asthma were also strongly linked to housing conditions, therefore, intervention to improve housing was essential to improve and maintain children's health [15].

E. Trade and Welfare [16-17]

It is the basic assumption that the change in social welfare when trade is allowed can be measured by the changes in producer and consumer surplus. Allowing good trade can increase social welfare in the sum of producer and consumer surplus.

This is because when a good is exported, suppliers gain and consumers lose, compared to the no trade position and when a good is imported, suppliers lose and consumers gain, compared to the no trade position. Since trade increases welfare of an economical system, welfare can be measured by the sum of producer and consumer surplus. It means social welfare is maximized at the competitive price and quantity for a good. Indeed, free trade is good for social welfare. However, there are some augments that should be mentioned: jobs argument, national defense argument, infant industry argument and unfair competition argument.

PUBLIC HEALTH CONCERN FOR PEOPLE IN THE RURAL COMMUNITY

A. Introduction

Public health is an important focus in medicine. Rural public health is a major part of public health. Rural public health must be viewed in the context of the entire system of health care [18-19]. Basically, rural people usually die of the same diseases as urban people, but often at higher rates. Deaths from accidents are also more prevalent in rural areas. Fewer resources to support public health initiatives in rural areas is common. The major aspects of rural public health include preventing epidemics, protecting against environmental hazards, preventing injuries, promoting healthy behaviors and responding to disasters [20-23]. Assuring quality and accessibility of health care for underserved populations are necessary.

It is a basic concept that if you've seen one rural community, you've seen one rural community. This means that there is a high variability among different settings and uniqueness in one setting. A good example is the different in ranging of health olympics among different countries. Japan is the country with the accepted best rural public health. Health care and economic development are integrally linked in rural areas. A concern on economical impact and rural public health will be discussed on this article.

B. Consideration on Public Health Policy

Rural health policy development focuses mainly on access issues [24-27]. The good public health policy generally doesn't different between distinction rural and urban. Good public health policy should be integral to ensuring the health of rural populations and accession to both public health and primary care professionals.

At present, the challenges in rural public health include poverty, inadequate transportation, remote distance, elder and economic decline. Increasing health care provider costs, shortages of providers, lack of facilities, decreasing federal and state subsidies, underprivileged groups in communes (pregnant, infant, elderly) and changing of consumers behavior to improper urban styles must be concerned.

Good rural public health policy should cover those themes. The important notes for rural area are trend of providing clinical services detracts from preventive activity, many dilemma clinical practices and provision of indigent care. The four main barriers; financial, geographic, organization and sociological factors, must be concerned. The main infrastructures to be concerned in rural public health include

1. leadership [28-29]

   The problem of leadership exists in many rural areas. It seems that good organization is still lack in many communes and this brings diminishing in rural representation. Fragmentation of public health programs are launched into villages. It is necessary to create correct perception of public health's role into the rural community. Development of strong public health leader is needed.

2. workforce preparedness [28-29]

   The certified public health employees are usually lack. Rural health usually faces a continuing problem of attracting and retaining the proper public health professionals. Although certificate or formal education in public health is available but there is only a few graduated worker. Many communities used the system of village health volunteer for running of public health system and this can lead to low quality project.

3. safety net provider support [29-30]

   Rural public health agencies caught lies on conflicting demands, population-based services versus supporting a safety net of personal health services. High degree providers, external to basic public health care system, can be seen in urban but it is hardly assessable and affordable by rural villagers. Over- and under- medical care are the problems for many communities.

4. managed care impact [31-32]

   Managed care has variable impact in rural areas. It has a strong potential to alter existing funding mechanisms. The systems appropriate for urban areas may not be appropriate for rural areas. Validation and selection need proper consideration.

5. Telecommunications [33-34]

   Telecommunications are the way for bringing new knowledge to the community. Since knowledge is the basement for attitude and practice, therefore, provision of knowledge by good telecommunication is needed.

   Most rural communities are still in need of telecommunications technology to take advantage of it. Stabilizing rural public health in communities requires starting with basic telecommunication equipment.

6. Funding [35]

   Public health funding is usually unstable. On the other hand, many funding are not necessarily tied to actual need. However, their own requirements, criteria, and expectations are usually poorly identified.

   Rural public health sections are usually received federal, state, and local funds.

C. Economic Development and Rural Health [24-25]

As previously mentioned, economic development and rural health are strongly correlated [26-27]. Strong linkage between rural development and health care improvement are proposed. It is necessary to using economic development to strengthen the rural health. Finding models to improving financial access is needed. When identifying the system of rural public health, it should cover all subsets (including hospitals, health care workers, nursing and protective care, home health, village health, public health, pharmacies and local politics). Focus must be systematized, broadening and in depth. How to balance the need of individual and the necessity is the main theme. Public understanding and expectation on population health, legal framework with system outcomes, broader social needs with appropriate limited financing system and balance of equity and choice between provider expectations and funding are the aims.

Health care is often overlooked. Limited employment in rural communities comparing to urban is a main factor for drainage of high skilled health care workers to the cities. Needs or health care consumers are rapid growing while quantity of providers is reducing. Similar to general economical principles, the more health care services are provided within rural communes, the greater the share of these moneys that return to the local economies. Demand for specialized, skilled workers coupled with push for cost reduction makes the hardness in balancing.

To know the present economical system is necessary for good planning of rural health policy [36]. Rural health care infrastructure must be carefully analyzed. Conducting community needs assessment planning processes including an analysis of the economics of the rural health care system are important basic requirement. These data can be used to stimulate the development of sound rural health policy in the macro-scale and it provides a common language between health, economic development, and local officers in micro- or local scale. It must be accepted the fact that less money is available for construction contrasting to future expansion. How to cope with the problem of fewer trained personnel with the trend of increasing retirement to private sections required urgent policy. Frequently communities have to manage themselves in "unsure" track. The objectives of such new projects are to improve health, improve quality of life, reduce time, reduce traveling and increase dignity. Hygiene and sanitation can be the monitoring markers.

Classification of Diseases

Disease is an overt disorder as previously mentioned. Thousands of diseases are listed in the medical documents. Classification of disease is required. There are many systems to classify diseases. In a common way, disease can be easily divided into infectious and non-infectious diseases. Infectious disease means any disease that is caused by infection. Infection is any condition that relates to the infective agents (bacteria, fungus, virus or parasite). Whereas non infectious disease is any disease that is not caused by infection, which is on the opposite side to infectious disease. Indeed, several other causes of disease, apart from infectious conditions, can be seen and usually problematic. Examples of infectious and non-infectious diseases are shown in Table 1.

In the same sense, two groups of diseases, communicable and non communicable diseases are also described. Communicable disease is usually equal to infectious disease while non communicable disease means non-infectious disease.

If classified by etiology, there will be many groups of disease. The main classified groups are

1. Trauma

   Trauma is a group of disease that is caused by injury. This is an important group of disease in the present. Accident is the leading cause of death for many countries. Trauma is usually sudden and acute. Prompt treatment is required. High mortality and morbidity can be seen.

2. Tumor

   Tumor is another important group of disease that becomes new problems for many countries. Tumor usually means cancer. However, some tumors are not cancerous. High mortality and morbidity can be seen especially in cases of cancer. Unluckily, exact causes of all cancers are not successfully detected. Focusing on cancer, no favorable treatment is available and there is a need for further research on this area.

3. Infection

   As previously noted, infectious disease means any disease that is caused by infection. This condition attacks millions of world population annually and it bring fatality to millions of world population.

4. Immune-related disease

   This is an interesting group of disease. Immune-related disease is a new focused. There are many new described diseases in the group of autoimmune disease. A long way for going is still left for diagnosis and treatment of immune-related diseases/

5. Intoxication

   Intoxication results from getting in toxins into the body by any methods (inhalation, skin contact, ingestion, injection and etc.) This is a problem and can be related to pollutant and environmental insults (for sure, there are also other groups of minor diseases that are not hereby mentioned).

Table 1. Examples of infectious and non-infectious diseases

Infectious diseases	Non infectious diseases
Rabies, typhoid fever, measles, ascariasis, filariasis, dengue fever, taeniasis	Diabetes mellitus, diabetes insipidus, Graves' disease, broken leg, burn, plubism, carbon monoxide intoxication

Using the model of holistic approach [37-40], disease can be seen in all categories: bio, psycho, social and spiritual. Irvine and Warber noted that incorporating the natural world into healthcare could provide health benefits and improve the design of healthcare facilities [41]. Irvine and Warber also indicated the importance of holistic approach [41]. Greaves et al. said that recent critiques of Western medicine focused mainly on the biopsychosocial model in relation to the former approach, but this could not deal adequately with the challenges that medicine currently related, because although it focused both the scientific and humanistic aspects of medicine it was not successful to harmonise them [42]. Therefore, harmonization is the important step for holistic treatment. Focus on each aspect will be hereby discussed.

1. Biological aspect

   As listed in the previous part, there are many biological disorders that can be seen in medicine. Those diseases are the core for classical treatment.

2. Pscyhological aspect

   Not only biological problem, psychological problem emerge in the present day. Pscychological stress can be seen by everyone in everyday. The increased incidence of psychological disorders at present brings psycholical diseases important topic in medicine. Abiodun said suggested that there was an urgent requirement to develop better collaboration between psychiatric and non-psychiatric physicians in clinical services, research and training at the primary, secondary and tertiary levels of health care [37].

3. Social and spiritual aspect

   Some diseases are directly related to local traditional. A so-called culture-bounded syndrome is mentioned.

Fade of Disease

Disorder or disease is an unhealthy condition of human beings. This is not a physiological condition. Fade of disease is a basic knowledge for all physicians. Any disease can result in many finalized outcomes. Without confounding factors, natural history of disease can be in these categories: self-limited or progression. With available treatment option, fade of disease include a) can be self-limited with or without treatment, b) can be cured if treated and cannot be cured if not treated, and c) cannot be cured with or without treatment. Examples of diseases that can be self-limited with or without treatment are cold and itching lesions from mosquito bite. Examples of diseases that can be cured if treated and cannot be cured if not treated are acute bacterial pneumonia and shigellosis. Examples of diseases that cannot be cured with or without treatment are rabies and poliomyelitis. With known fade of disease, any disease can be proper managed. This is helpful for classification and policy planning for preventive purpose. Due to simple rational, diseases that can be self-limited with or without treatment might not receive high priority but diseases that can be cured if treated and cannot be cured if not treated should receive the highest priority and selected group to receive treatment [43-45]. However, this does not mean that other diseases apart from the group that that can be cured if treated and cannot be cured if not treated require no treatment and neglected. Despite the group that cannot be cured with or without treatment supportive and symptomatic treatments should be provided to relief the pain and unhappiness of the affected patients. This is the basic rule of medicine.

Considering the phase of treatment, there can be several phases. Early treatment means treatment at early stage of disease. This is called as prompt treatment and can be secondary prevention. This is focused in the present day. It also shifted to the treatment before disease or pre-symptomatic treatment. Late treatment means treatment at late stage. This is usually related to high mortality and morbidity. This is not wanted. Another meaning can be the rehabilitation which is the tertiary prevention to limit the extension of disability.

How to Treat?

A basic principle of physician is treatment. However, it must reconfirm for the roles of physicians which include diagnosis, treatment and prevention. The treatment process is usually the final step. The treatment is usually a following process of diagnosis. Without diagnosis, treatment cannot and should not be performed. Although the definitive diagnosis is not derived the provisional diagnosis by clinical appearance of the patients must be derived before planning any treatments. Therefore, it is necessary to talk about diagnosis in medicine. Diagnosis of any diseases should be done after the complete history taking and physical examination. An important process is to perform a complete systemic review focusing on all organ system of the patients. Laboratory diagnosis is the following tool for help confirm diagnosis or theoretical thought of clinical summary from history taking and physical examination. Several laboratory investigations are available at present and should be carefully selected for proper usage. To rationally select, the physicians must have good basic knowledge on clinical pathology. Laboratory medicine is a requirement course for all undergraduate medical students.

When the completeness of diagnosis step is done, it is the major role of the next step, treatment or therapy. The basic concept for treatment is a) getting rid of the etiological factor or cause of disease and b) limiting and recovering of the destructive part due to the disease. This concept can be applied for all kinds of diseases. It is a basic and good solution to the query how to perform a treatment. Getting rid of etiological factor can be done by many methods especially for medical and surgical procedures. Similar processes can be used for limitation and recovery of pathological findings from disease. Medical or surgical procedures might be selected.

As a case study, the author will demonstrate the case of case bacterial pneumonia. What is the proper treatment? The first aim to get rid of etiological factor will be firstly focused. The etiology due to the given diagnosis is due to bacterial infection. Bacteria is accepted as the etiology of this disease. This can be diagnosed by method of basic microbiology test. Sputum examination might reveal Gram's positive bacteria. If there is any evidences from laboratory examinations as described, the outcome of treatment can better warranted. The treatment for getting rid of the pathogen is antibiotic treatment. Penicillin might be administered. For the second purpose to limit and recover, symptomatic and supportive treatments such as antipyretic drug and intravenous fluid administration can be used. Another case of dog bite will be hereby further discussed. The first aim to get rid of the etiology is the management of the wound because the wound is the thing that brings the patient to visit the clinic. Management of wound by wound dressing is the first step. For second purpose for limitation and recovery, tetanus toxoid, rabies vaccination, oral antibiotic and analgesic drug can be given. These were all further prescribed after primary wound caring. It can be seen that limitation of disease in this case study can be also accepted as the prevention based on preventive medicine. Prompt treatment is the rule of secondary prevention. Finally, the last case of ovarian tumor will be mentioned and hereby discussed. To get rid of the cause of disease or tumor, a surgical procedure namely oophorectomy can be selected. This is the removal of the problematic mass at ovary. For limitation and recovery, the symptomatic and supportive care, especially for post operative period must be given and planned. In addition, it there is later additional diagnosis from following up laboratory investigations such as cancerous finding from histopathology of surgical specimen, additional treatment as chemotherapy should be set. These examples might be helpful for the reader to generate the idea and better understand of the concept of treatment in medicine.

Finally, the author would like to mention for the ethics for medical treatment.

Similar to diagnosis, different in medical treatment can be seen. An important widely discussed problem at present is "double standard [48]." The problem can be seen in medicine and can bring the threat to medical society. The problems are mainly due to overtreatment or refusing for treatment because of socioeconomic problem of the patient. This has to be avoided. The principle of "first do no harm" must be used.

References

[1] Mata LJ. The environment of the malnourished child. *Basic Life Sci.* 1976;7:45-66.

[2] Abel-Smith B. Health economics in developing countries. *J Trop Med Hyg.* 1989;92:229-41.

[3] den Hartog AP. Eat well and stay healthy. Changing perspectives on good nutrition, *Ned Tijdschr Tandheelkd.* 1995;102:419-22.

[4] Howell N. Demographic anthropology. *Annu Rev Anthropol.* 1986;15:219-46.

[5] Gonzalez-Barranco J, Rios-Torres JM. Early malnutrition and metabolic abnormalities later in life. *Nutr Rev.* 2004 Jul;62(7 Pt 2):S134-9.

[6] Battistini NC, Malavolti M, Poli M, Pietrobelli A. Growth: healthy status and active food model in pediatrics. *Int J Obes* (Lond). 2005 Sep;29 Suppl 2:S14-8.

[7] Hickson M. Malnutrition and ageing. Postgrad Med J. 2006 Jan;82(963):2-8.

[8] Smith GD. Life-course approaches to inequalities in adult chronic disease risk. *Proc Nutr Soc.* 2007 May;66(2):216-36.

[9] Szpak A. Does Polish public health strategy give consideration to the manner of nutrition and its consequences for health? *Wiad Lek.* 2002;55 Suppl 1(Pt 2):927-34.

[10] Hunt SM, McEwen J, McKenna SP. Social inequalities and perceived health. *Eff Health Care.* 1985;2(4):151-60.

[11] Townsend P. Toward equality in health through social policy. *Int J Health Serv.* 1981;11(1):63-75.

[12] Aoyama H. Background and prospects of the Community Health Act] *Nippon Eiseigaku Zasshi.* 1996 Feb;50(6):1026-35.

[13] Hill P. Ethics and health systems research in 'post'-conflict situations. *Dev World Bioeth.* 2004 Dec;4(2):139-53.

[14] Kaminskas R, Darulis Z. Peculiarities of medical sociology: application of social theories in analyzing health and medicine. *Medicina* (Kaunas). 2007;43(2):110-7.

[15] Chaudhuri N. Interventions to improve children's health by improving the housing environment. *Rev Environ Health.* 2004 Jul-Dec;19(3-4):197-222.

[16] Heath SE. Challenges and options for animal and public health services in the next two decades. *Rev Sci Tech.* 2006 Apr;25(1):403-19.

[17] Holden C. Privatization and trade in health services: a review of the evidence. *Int J Health Serv.* 2005;35(4):675-89.

[18] The politics of public sector change. *Aust Fam Physician.* 2003 May;32(5):373-5.

[19] Field JE, Peck E. Public-private partnerships in healthcare: the managers' perspective. *Health Soc Care Community.* 2003 Nov;11(6):494-501.

[20] Pratt DS. Occupational health and the rural worker: agriculture, mining, and logging. *J Rural Health.* 1990 Oct;6(4):399-417.

[21] Handel DA, Hedges JR; SAEM IOM Task Force. Improving rural access to emergency physicians. *Acad Emerg Med.* 2007 Jun;14(6):562-5.

[22] Dummer TJ, Cook IG. Exploring China's rural health crisis: processes and policy implications. *Health Policy.* 2007 Sep;83(1):1-16.

[23] Singh R, Singh A, Servoss TJ, Singh G. Prioritizing threats to patient safety in rural primary care. *J Rural Health.* 2007 Spring;23(2):173-8.

[24] Forde K, Malley A. Privatisation in health care: theoretical considerations, current trends and future options. *Aust Health* Rev. 1992;15(3):269-77.

[25] Kizito NB. The politics of reconstructing the health sector and the informal health market: non-established links. *Sante.* 1997 Nov-Dec;7(6):423-4.

[26] Wright DD. Recent rural health research. *J Community Health.* 1976 Fall;2(1):60-72.

[27] Barrett LT. The need for a regional focus in rural health services. *Public Health Rep.* 1975 Jul-Aug;90(4):349-56.

[28] Kelley ML, MacLean MJ. I want to live here for rest of my life. The challenge of case management for rural seniors. *J Case Manag.* 1997 Winter;6(4):174-82.

[29] Oosterhoff DD, Cand SJ, Rowell M. Shared leadership: the freedom to do bioethics. *HEC Forum.* 2004 Dec;16(4):297-316

[30] Bullock S, Schou P, Sexton W, Stuart P. A critical role. Roundtable discussion. *Mod Healthc.* 2007 Nov 5;37(44):24-7.

[31] Basu J, Friedman B, Burstin H. Preventable hospitalization and medicaid managed care: does race matter? *J Health Care Poor Underserved.* 2006 Feb;17(1):101-15.

[32] Ahern M, McCoy V. Effects of payment changes on urgent/emergent admissions in rural and urban communities. *J Rural Health.* 1993 Spring;9(2):120-8.

[33] Morosini P. Telemedicine: past, present and future. *Recenti Prog Med.* 2006 Nov;97(11):647-51.

[34] Jennett PA, Gagnon MP, Brandstadt HK. Preparing for success: readiness models for rural telehealth. *J Postgrad Med.* 2005 Oct-Dec;51(4):279-85.

[35] Straub LA. Financing rural health and medical services. *J Rural Health.* 1990 Oct;6(4):467-84.

[36] Pate JA. New hope for rural health. *Tex Med.* 1991 Feb;87(2):30-2.

[37] Abiodun OA. The need for a holistic approach to patient care. *East Afr Med J.* 1991 Jan;68(1):25-8

[38] Thomas SA, Hargett T. Mental health care: a collaborative, holistic approach. *Holist Nurs Pract.* 1999 Jan;13(2):78-85.

[39] Vreeland B. Bridging the gap between mental and physical health: a multidisciplinary approach. *J Clin Psychiatry.* 2007;68 Suppl 4:26-33.

[40] Gordon JS. Holistic medicine and mental health practice: toward a new synthesis. *Am J Orthopsychiatry.* 1990 Jul;60(3):357-70.

[41] Irvine KN, Warber SL. Greening healthcare: practicing as if the natural environment really mattered. *Altern Ther Health Med.* 2002 Sep-Oct;8(5):76-83.

[42] Greaves D. Reflections on a new medical cosmology. *J Med Ethics.* 2002 Apr;28(2):81-5.

[43] Maciosek MV, Coffield AB, McGinnis JM, Harris JR, Caldwell MB, Teutsch SM, Atkins D, Richland JH, Haddix A. Methods for priority setting among clinical preventive services. *Am J Prev Med.* 2001 Jul;21(1):10-9.

[44] Maciosek MV, Edwards NM, Coffield AB, Flottemesch TJ, Nelson WW, Goodman MJ, Solberg LI. Priorities among effective clinical preventive services: methods. *Am J Prev Med.* 2006 Jul;31(1):90-6.

[45] Cho W, Lee S, Kang HY, Kang M. Setting national priorities for quality assessment of health care services in Korea. *Int J Qual Health Care.* 2005 Apr;17(2):157-65.

[46] Bostrom N. In defense of posthuman dignity. *Bioethics.* 2005 Jun;19(3):202-14.

[47] Cox P. Codes of medical ethics and the exportation of less-than-standard care. *Int J Appl Philos.* 1999 Fall;13(2):177-85.

[48] Ackerman AB. No double standard for patient care. *Am J Dermatopathol.* 1984 Aug;6(4):411.

Chapter II

NANOTHERAPY

INTRODUCTION TO NANOSCIENCE [1-7]

Nanotechnology is a modern technology covering to management, construction, synthesis of devices in atomic or molecular level that has its the size between, 1 and 100 nanometers. The nanodevice has its special function in physical, chemical and biological aspect that can be adapted for usage. Nanotechnology is the application of knowledge on nanoscience [8-10]. Nanoscience is a modern science covering on the natural fact of nanolevel conditions. Nanoscience focuses on three main scientific areas: physical, chemical and biological sciences. The main fundamental knowledge for the beginner in nanoscience is what nanolevel is. "Nano" is a modern scientific work describing for the 10^{-9} level. The nanolevel is minuteder or fewer than microlevel (micro = 10^{-6}). Nanotechnologies can assist practitioner diagnosis at the single-cell and molecule levels, and some can be adapted in current molecular diagnostic methods, such as biochips [11]. Nanoparticles, such as gold nanoparticles, silver nanoparticles and quantum dots, are the most broadly used, but various other nanotechnological devices for manipulation at the nanoscale as well as nanobiosensors are also promising for potential clinical applications [11]. In conclusion, nanotechnologies will expand the borders of current molecular diagnostics and assist in point-of-care diagnostics, integration of diagnostics with therapeutics, and modern construction of personalized medicine [11]. Jain mentioned for the emerging role of advances in biochip and microarray technologies in the modern construction of personalized medicine [12]. Jain proposed that biochips such as GeneChip, CYP450, electrochemical biochips, protein biochips, microfluidic biochips and nanotechnology-based biochips played a significant role in molecular diagnostics, and their application in point-of-care diagnosis is expected to facilitate the modern construction of personalized medicine [12]. Although the potential diagnostic applications are wildly expanded, the most important current applications are limited in the areas of biomarker discomuch, cancer diagnosis, and determination of infectious pathogens [11].

Why "Nanotherapy"? [12-16]

Treatment is an important medical activity. Although it is accepted that prevention is better than treatment therapy for already presented disorder is necessary. Therapy can be either specific or symptomatic treatment aiming at curative or minimize suffer of the illed subject. Modern construction of treatment has been continuous for years and nanotherapy is a modern advent is medical treatment and becomes a modern hope in medicine. At present, it reveals that there are still several limited sides of old-kindd treatment. The specificity of treatment in old-kindd therapy is a focus. It is accepted that old-kindd therapy is limited in site and size of treatment. Access to the right site is the key for the most powerful treatment. It cannot be repeated that the best connection is the connection at the real problematic issueatic site. This is the way of thought of medical treatment. Indeed Retail hers proposed for the way of thought of magic bullet since the nineteenth century [17-19]. This way of thought is the focus for pharmacological treatment at present. The best case study is the case of chemotherapy. In the old-kindd chemotherapy, lack of good site specificity brings many complications; destroying of non cancerous cells [20-22]. For size specific, the best case study is the concern on surgical wound [23-25]. Now, the way of thought of present surgery is the least injured practical method. This way of thought is also corresponding to the basic medical rule "First do no harm [26-30]".

The answer to the query "How can we search the site and size specific therapy?" has been searched for years. Luckily, due to the advanced nanobiotechnology, the answer reveals to be reached. The core way of thought of nanotechnology is the "small". In one sense, small means specific: focus on a limited scoped site and size. In addition, due to rule of nanomaterial, including surface area effect will quainter effect, application of nanomaterials as modern supplement alien to improve old-kindd therapeutic protocol can be much valuable. In this chapter, the details on advanced nanotherapy will be summarized and presented.

Nanosurgery and Nanodentistry

Neurosurgery is the modern way of thought in surgical medicine [31-32]. As previously mentioned, minuted wound is a focus of present surgery. The way of thought is that minuted surgical wound means minuted alignment of blood loss and minimization of intraoperative and post operative complication. Minuted wound also reduce the postoperative hospitalized period for the illed subject. However, the real nanosurgery for human beings has rarely been reached. There are some advents in eye surgery. Femtosecond laser pulses, emitted from lasers working in the near infrared, based on multiphoton effects permit both imaging and laser effects to be generated which are in the submicron range and which do not cause collateral destruction is available [33]. Similar to nanosurgery, application of nanobiotechnology for nanodentistry [34] can be early reported as the modern construction of many instruments and devices. Nanotechnology also has a significant relationship in dentistry materials.

Gene Therapy and Nanobiotechnology

Gene therapy is the advanced therapeutic way of thought at present. By definition, gene therapy implies to local or systemic administration of a nucleic acid construct that can prevent, treat and even cure diseases by changing the expression of genes that are corresponding for the pathological condition. Gene therapy involves gene manipulation and transfer. A number of polymer-based synthetic systems, or 'vectors', have been developed to entice cells to use exogenous DNA [35]. This therapy is the hope for treatment of presently non curable diseases. Gene-delivery systems usually include a carrier system which both protects the gene expression plasmid and permits its extracellular and intracellular transportation [36]. Viruses are used in most of the clinical tests today; however, they do have important drawbacks, therefore, non-viral vectors based on lipids, water-soluble polycations, other non-condensing polymers and nano- or microparticles/capsules have been proposed [36]. Nanobiotechnology can be adapted for the complex gene therapy process. At present, both biodegradable and non-biodegradable inorganic particles can be successfully fabricated in the nano-scale with the attributes of binding DNA, internalizing across the plasma membrane and lastly releasing it in the cytoplasm for final expression of a protein [37]. In addition to the old-kindd system (intravenous injection), modern construction of polymer-based nanoparticle technologies for oral gene therapy is ongoing [38].

Stem Cell Therapy, Tissue Engineering and Nanobiotechnology

Stem cell therapy is another advanced therapeutic way of thought. It is adapted for treatment of many diseases especially for congenital defects and malignancies. The best case studies of nanobiotechnology application in stem cell therapy can be seen in nanohenatology [39-42]. Tissue engineering is another advanced biotechnology that is valuable for regenerative medicine [43]. Basically, cross-linking and cross-bridging are highly versatile methods of creating composite protein structures with desired mechanical properties such as deformation endurance, elasticity, extensibility, and stability under intensive and repetitive sheering forces [44]. The nanomaterials can be used as structural cross-linking and cross-bridging polymers for the modern generated tissues. With the ability to form nano-fibrous structures, a drive to mimic the extracellular matrix and form scaffolds that are an artificial extracellular matrix suitable for tissue formation has begun [45-46]. Simth and Ma proposed that the nano-fibrous scaffolds attempted to mimic collagen, a natural extracellular matrix component, and could potentially provide a better environment for tissue formation in tissue engineering systems [45]. Murugan and Ramakrishna noted that scaffolds played a pivotal role in supporting the cells to accommodate and guided their growth into a specific tissue; therefore, designing scaffolds that are favorable to cellular growth was importance [47]. Murugan and Ramakrishna also said that electrospinning was a straightforward, cost-effective, and versatile technique that could be adapted for the fabrication of nano-featured scaffolds suitable for tissue engineering and it bringed many advantages over conventional scaffold methodologies [47].

Nanobiosensor implant should also be mentioned. Nanobiosensor implant is an application of nanobiodievice. At present, it is accepted that it is probable to implant a much minuted, nanoscale, biodevice into the human body. The nanobiosensor implant can be valuable for treatment aiming at physiological response to the rhythmic change in human body. The best case study is the case of diabetes mellitus, which is an endocrine disorder [48]. Basically, the diabetes mellitus is the disease with insulin, pancreatic hormone, disorder. The treatment must match with the daily physiological rhythmic change of insulin in the human beings.

APPLICATION BY NANOPHARMACOLOGY

Steady progress in the identification of human pharmacogenetic variants and modern discoveries of disease susceptibility genes makes the old notion of one disease/one drug untenable [49]. The present way of thought of pharmacology is highly selective pharmacological therapy. This way of thought has been proposed for centuries. This way of thought was firstly propagated by Paul Ehrlich. The best case study of magic bullet way of thought is adapted for cancer therapy [50-51]. There is a great need for more specific focusing of chemotherapeutic agents, but modern construction of specific therapy will be hard in light of the barriers which separate a tumor from the vasculature, tumor cell heterogeneity and instability, technological advances necessary for drug delivery design and introduction into the clinic and mechanisms for assessment of efficacy [52]. However, Kreuter et al. noted that behavioral and social strategies will not come in the form of pre-packaged, easily exported "magic bullets," complete with efficacy estimates, for the prevention and control of selected cancers [53].

Nanotechnology is the modern hope to lead us directly to the magic bullet [54-56]. Indeed, the technology is expected to create innovations and play a crucial role in various biomedical applications, not only in drug delivery, but also in molecular imaging, biomarkers and biosensors [57]. Focus-specific drug therapy and methods for early diagnosis of pathologies are the priority research areas where nanotechnology would play a vital role [57]. During the past 30 years, the explosive growth of nanotechnology has burst into challenging innovations in pharmacology, the main input being the ability to perform temporal and spatial site-specific delivery [54-56]. This has led to some marketed compounds through the last decade [54].

Introducing foreign bodies into the complex machinery of the human body is, however, a great and humbling challenge [58]. In order for nanobiology to reach its full potential, a means to alter the properties of nanoparticles, as expressed in the human body, in a predictable manner is needed [58]. Computer-aided methods are the natural choice to speed up the modern construction of these technologies [59]. In silico nanobio-design is important technique. The important step for in silico drug design will be further reported.

A. Genome Sequence Analysis

Genome sequence analysis is valuable for searching of modern drugs, especially for infectious diseases. The availability of a complete microbial genome sequence in 1995 brought the originating of a genomic era that has permited medical scientists to change the paradigm and approach vaccine modern construction originating from genomic information [60]. The whole-genome perspective is expected to provide an instrumental contribution to drug and vaccine modern construction, particularly to focus those pathogens for which the traditional approaches have failed so far [61]. Combining pathogen genome sequences with the host and vector genome sequences is promising to be a robust method for the identification of host-pathogen interactions. In additional, comparative sequencing of related species, especially of organisms used as model systems in the study of the disease, is beginning to realize its potential in the identification of genes that are involved in evasion of the host immune response [62]. These data are all valuable in drug and vaccine modern construction [63].

B. Microarrays

Identification of an immune response correlate for protection against pathogen would greatly facilitate the rational modern construction of an effective vaccine. However, detecting such a correlate has been a daunting task. DNA microarray technology is a modern and powerful tool that permits the simultaneous analysis of a large number of nucleic acid hybridization experiments in a rapid and efficient fashion [64]. An advantage of microarray technology is that it can assist researchers to better define and understand the expression profile of a given genokind associated with disease, adverse effects from exposure to certain stimuli, or the ability to understand or predict immune responses to specific antigens [64]. The modern construction of DNA microarray technology a decade ago brought the establishment of functional genomics as one of the most active and successful scientific disciplines at present [65].

C. Proteomics Approach and High-Throughput Cloning

Despite the increasing availability of genome sequences from many human pathogens, the production of complete proteomes remains at a bottleneck. Traditionally, the production of a recombinant protein requires a preliminary cloning step of the focus gene into an expression vector before evaluating its cellular expression [66-67]. Among current methods, site-specific recombination cloning techniques, which eliminate the use of restriction endonucleases and ligase, bring several advantages in the context of high throughput practical methods [67]. Rapid and highly efficient, the recombinational cloning technology is largely used for structural genomics and functional proteomics [66-67]. High-throughput approaches for gene cloning and expression require the modern construction of modern, nonstandard tools for use by molecular biologists and biochemists [68]. High-throughput

PCR recombination cloning and expression platform has been developed that permits hundreds of genes to be batch-processed by using basic laboratory practical methods [69]. The derived data can be valuable for drug and vaccine modern construction.

D. Bioinformatics Database Tools and Computational Vaccinology

Several advance bioinfomatics have been launched for a few years and these database tools are valuable for vaccine modern constructions. Huge amounts of data are produced by genomics and proteomics projects and large-scale screening of pathogen-host and antigen-host interactions. For vaccine discomuch, one can "mine" the genomic sequence for potential surface focus using various algorithms, characterize these gene focus, and produce primers for cloning, all before one enters the wet laboratory [70]. Both, predictions and the interpretation of experiments rely on existing information in the literature which is mostly manually extracted [71]. These can be addressed well by quantitative experimental and theoretical biophysical techniques, and particularly by methods from drug design [72]. Databases and data mining, the two principal weapons at the disposal of the in silico drug search. Future modern construction will also include systemic models of drug and vaccine responses [73]. The common in silico methods include databases, quantitative structure-activity relationships, similarity searching, pharmacophores, homology models and other molecular modeling, machine learning, data mining, network analysis tools and data analysis tools that use a computer [74-79]. Such methods have seen frequent use in the discomuch and optimization of novel molecules with affinity to a focus, the clarification of absorption, distribution, metabolism, excretion and toxicity properties as well as physicochemical characterization [74-79]. More details can be seen in the chapter of nanoinformatics. Jain said that the nanotechnology can assist drug searching to reach the state of personalized medicine, which implied magic bullet [80]. Morrow et al. said that site-specific focused drug delivery and personalized medicine were just a few way of thoughts that were on the horizon [81]. In conclusion, nanotechnology is proved to be much important for future personalized medicine and systems biology [82,83]. Indeed, nanotechnology realizes the advantages of naturally occurring biological macromolecules and their building-block nature for design [84]. Frequently, assembly originates with the choice of a good molecule that is synthetically optimized towards the desired shape from the previously reported nanobio-design [84]. However, Tsai et al. proposed another alternative originating with a pre-specified nanostructure shape, selecting candidate protein building blocks from a library and mapping them onto the shape and, lastly, testing the stability of the construct [84].

Nanotechnology and Drug Delivery

In addition to designing, drug delivery is another focus of interest [85-91]. Application of nanotechnology for drug delivery is accepted in pharmacology. At present, nanoparticles are considered to have the potential as novel intravascular or cellular probes for both diagnostic (imaging) and therapeutic purposes (drug/gene delivery), which is expected to generate innovations and play a crucial role in medicine [87]. The application of nanotechnology on drug delivery can be seen in four important areas as controlled release of drug, prolongation of drug life-time, acceleration of drug absorption and drug focusing.

A. Controlled Release of Drug

To convey a sufficient dose of drug to the lesion, suitable carriers of drugs are necessary [92]. Conventional dosage means, such as oral delivery or injection, are the predominant routes for drug delivery [93]. The main drawbacks of these kinds of dosages consist essentially in a limited control of the drug delivery rate and of the focus area [93]. Nanoparticle carriers have important potential applications for the administration of therapeutic molecules without the quoted problematic issue [92]. Nanoparticles are important controlled drug delivery devices [92].

B. Prolongation of Drug Life-Time

Prolongation of drug life-time is another application of nanomaterial in drug delivery. For case study, the modification of drug with water soluble nanopolymer can assist hold the drug in the vessel. Zhou et al. mentioned that biodegradable colloidal nano-micelles was a novel focusing drug delivery and controlled release system, which could prolong the biological half-life and lighten the toxicity of chemotherapeutant, meanwhile, present fine biocompatibility [94]. In 2006, Pattani et al. reported a work on modern construction and comparative anti-microbial evaluation of lipid nanoparticles and nanoemulsion of Polymyxin B [95]. Pattani et al. reported that the developed lipid nanoparticles and nanoemulsion were promising delivery vectors for the anti-microbial drugs and lipid nanoparticles could give an initial as well as sustained effect while the nanoemulsion was capable of exerting potent effect for a shorter period of time [95]. In 2007, Liu et al. reported another work on fate of unimers and micelles of a poly(ethylene glycol)-block-poly(caprolactone) copolymer in mice following intravenous administration [96]. Liu et al. reported that the hydrophobic and semi-crystalline nature of the poly(ethylene glycol)-b-poly(caprolactone) core imparted a high degree of kinetic stability to this micelle system [96]. In 2004, Li et al. done another interesting study to investigate the preparation technique,shape characteristics, and drug releasing characteristics in vivo of 5-FU loaded core-shell kind nanoparticles which were made by biodegradable amphiphlic poly (ethylene glycol)-poly (gamma-benzyl-L-glutamate)(PEG-PBLG) [97].

Li et al. found that the 5-FU/PEG-PBLG nano-micelles could change the pharmacokinetics of 5-FU, prolonging the circulation time in vivo and mad a slow release [97].

C. Acceleration of Drug Absorption

Nanoparticle can assist acceleration of drug absorption by decreasing biological barriers of cells and tissues. Cevc said that colloids from an aqueous suspension could cross the skin barrier only through hydrophilic pathways [98]. Cevc also proposed that various colloids had a different ability to do this by penetrating narrow pores of fixed size in the skin, or the relevant nano-pores in barriers modeling the skin [98]. Liposome is a broadly used nanoparticle for acceleration of drug absorption. Fang said that classic liposomes were of little value as carriers for drug delivery by the skin because they did not penetrate it deeply [99]. Fang also mentioned that only specially designed liposomes had been shown to be capable of achieving increased delivery [99]. Basically, manipulation of the physical properties of drug delivery system provides improved control over the pharmacokinetics and pharmacodynamics of the encapsulated drugs relative to free drugs [100]. Liposomes can act as sustained release delivery system and manipulation of properties such as, liposome diameter, drug release rate, bioavailability and dosing schedule can significantly impact the therapeutic outcome of the liposomal drugs [100].

D. Drug Focusing

Nanoparticle can assist drug focusing by drug focus recognition. Over the last few years, nano-structures have been developed in order to improve the efficiency and the specificity of drug action [101]. Their minuted size permits them to be injected intravenously in order to reach focus tissues [101]. This application is previously discussed in the way of thought of magic bulleting. It is broadly used for anticancer drug. Selective delivery to solid tumor sites can be done by utilizing increased permeability and retention effect of solid tumor sites [102]. Essential factors of carriers systems based on this mechanism is size and chemical character of carriers [102]. To design a favorable nanoparticle that is most suitable for drug focusing, layer-by-layer assembly can be used as a versatile bottom-up nanofabrication technique [103].

There are many nanomaterials that are presently adapted for drug delivery. However, the most broadly used ones are aptamer, liposome and dendrimer.

A. Aptamer

Numerous nucleic acid ligands, also termed decoys or aptamers, have been developed during the past 15 years that can prevent the activity of many pathogenic proteins [104]. ptamers may prove valuable in the treatment of a broad variety of human disorders, including infectious diseases, cancer, and cardiovascular disease.

B. Liposome

Liposome is an spherical shape nanopolymer and its main composition of liposome is sugar and protein that can act as the receptor (more details can be seen in another chapter on this book). The good characteristic of liposome can assist accelerate of drug absorption as previously mentioned. In many cases liposomal drugs are administered by the bloodstream [105]. The stability in the bloodstream, clearance, and biodistribution are dependent on the composition, size, and charge of the liposomes [105]. Rigid, minuted-size (100-200 nm) liposomes tend to be retained in the blood without degradation [105]. There are many recent advent on liposome technology. Long-circulating liposome is a good case study [105]. Three kinds of functional long-circulating liposomes are available at present, namely, thermosensitive liposomes for delivering macromolecules, pH-sensitive liposomes for the cytosolic delivery of encapsulated materials, and reticuloendothelial system - avoiding liposomes for the passive focusing to tumor tissues [106]. In addition, it has become increasingly evident that tissues utilize specific localization of enzymes to perform certain tasks, often associated with various kinds of tissue remodeling [107]. The ubiquitous presence of such enzymes, along with their specific localizations, provides an ideal opportunity to elicit specific delivery by an enzyme-triggered mechanism [107].

C. Dendrimer

Dendriner is a synthesized nanopolymer with dendrogram, three-branched style, structure (more details can be seen in another chapter on this book). Dendrimer can significantly improve pharmacokinetic and pharmacodynamic properties of low molecular weight and protein-based therapeutic agents [108]. Furthermore, fluorescent antibodies and imaging contrast agents can be bound to these modern polymers and the resulting complexes can be used for analyzing biological fluids and for diagnosis [108].

D. Transfersome

Transfersomes (Idea AG) are a form of elastic or deformable vesicle, which were first introduced in the early 1990s [109]. Elasticity can be generated by incorporation of an edge activator in the lipid bilayer structure [109]. The main composition of these vesicles is soya phosphatidyl choline incorporating sodium cholate and a minuted concentration of ethanol [109]. Transfersomes can be adapted in a non-occluded method to the skin and have been shown to permeate through the stratum corneum lipid lamellar parts as a result of the hydration or osmotic force in the skin [110].

NANOVACCINOLOGY

Similar to nanopharmacology, computer-aided methods are the basic choice to develop the modern construction in nanovaccinology. Basically, vaccine modern construction includes detecting the epitope of focused protein, modern construction of recombinant and test for its efficacy. Routinely, this process originates from in vitro researches to in vivo researches (from animal model to human clinical studies). In addition to the old-kindd immunological technique, with advent in bioinformatics, modern construction of modern cancer vaccine can be done by advanced in silico techniques. The important steps for vaccine modern construction will be further explained and discussed.

A. Detecting epitope

To find a peptide candidate for a vaccine, the originating point is to find proper epitpes. Different practical methods for epitope mapping are available at present [111]. It should be noted that synthetic peptide vaccines aiming at the induction of a protective response against malignant diseases are broadly tested but despite their success in animal models they do not yet live up to their promise in humans [112]. Mapping for probable epitopes reveals to be a hard step. The evidence accumulating from many recent studies points to a broader range of focus recognized than previously expected, in terms of both numbers and characteristics of the focused antigens [113]. Also, multiple studies report a substantial variation in the focused recognized in different human individuals [113]. To solve the problematic issue of heterogenicity, many modern computational tools are developed for detecting of probable candidate vaccine epitopes. Prediction of both T cell and B cell epitopes for further cancer vaccine modern construction can be easily done. Nanoinformatics can assist these processes.

B. Modern construction of modern vaccine recombinant

Modern construction of modern vaccine recombinant from alternative epitope is the next step. This can be done based on rule of artificial genetic recombinant. To develop modern genetic recombinant, advanced gene delivery and transfer technique can be used. Of several techniques, gene transfer by virus or transfection in the most broadly used. The nanoparticle can assist gene delivery.

C. Testing for modern vaccine efficacy

Testing for modern vaccine efficacy is the final step of vaccine modern construction. This can be done as the reported process in the heading of research into cancer vaccine. Clinical tests should be done before real expansion of the modern vaccine. In order to reduce the long step of clinical test, the application of advanced medical informatics technology, gene ontology [114], can assist predict the function or phenotypic expression of modern developed vaccine.

D. Adaptation of the presented vaccine techniques by nanotechnology

In addition to searching and generation for modern vaccine, adaptation of the presented vaccine techniques by nanotechnology can be done. The adaptation makes use of nanoparticles mostly for delivery purposed.

ETHICAL ASPECT OF NANOTECHNOLOGY

A successful method for control of scientific technology is ethical control. It is accepted that good ethical control stranded accompany scientific activity. Increasingly, risks from new and emerging technologies are being controled at the international level, although governments and private experts are only beginning to consider the appropriate international responses to nanotechnology [115]. There are many aspects of ethical concern on new technology. The first basic principle is that it is necessary to until that the new technology is a real good technology. This also implies that it is a safe technology and dies not have side effects. This fact is once discussed in the environmental aspect of nanotechnology in the previous part of this chapter. It should be noted that since the nanoparticles is still under double-times for its safety and there is a possibility for its side effects, there is a need to set a street control program of the nanomaterial synthesized laboratory. The syntheses labiality must be accredited and useful for the safety student, which unit includes physic bio-chemo items. Concept of ethics in laboratory medicine can be applied for nanotechnology [116-117]. The concept can also be adapted for nano-, bio-, info-, and cogno- convergence technologies [118]. Sententia et al. proposed that scientists required analytical models that protect values of personhood at the heart of a functional democracy-values that help, as much as possible, for individual decision-making, despite transformations in understanding and ability to manipulate cognitive processes [118]. Sententia et al. stated that addressing cognitive enhancement from the legal and ethical notion of cognitive liberty could bring a powerful tool for assessing and encouraging nano-bio-info-cogno developments [118]. It can be said that nanoethics is a new field of ethical inquiry [119]. The important topics on nanoethics will be further detailed.

A. Concern on nanotechnology research

Similar to any biomedical research, the main question for nanotechnology research is "How should the dignity of people participating in nanomedicine research trials be respected?". The two main portions to be considered is the protection of individuals involving the the nanotechnology research. Protection of individuals should be applied to both health care and medical research. The second concern is on informed consent. This is the basic requirement in biomedical research. However, it may be hard to provide proper information concerning a proposed nanotechnology research because there is no confirmation on the safety of nanoparticles as previously noted. Initiatives should be taken to enhance information exchange between research ethics committees in different settings. Although there are many ways for applied nanobiotechnology, health care considerations must be met first priority [120].

REFERENCES

[1] Kane RS, Stroock AD. Nanobiotechnology: protein-nanomaterial interactions. *Biotechnol Prog*. 2007 Mar-Apr;23(2):316-9.

[2] Medvedeva NV, Ipatova OM, Ivanov IuD, Drozhzhin AI, Archakov AI. Nanobiotechnology and nanomedicine. *Biomed Khim*. 2006 Nov-Dec;52(6):529-46.

[3] Blattler T, Huwiler C, Ochsner M, Stadler B, Solak H, Voros J, Grandin HM Nanopatterns with biological functions. *J Nanosci Nanotechnol*. 2006 Aug;6(8):2237-64.

[4] Groneberg DA, Giersig M, Welte T, Pison U. Nanoparticle-based diagnosis and therapy. *Curr Drug Focus*. 2006 Jun;7(6):643-8.

[5] Jain KK. The role of nanobiotechnology in drug discomuch. *Drug Discov Today*. 2005 Nov 1;10(21):1435-42.

[6] Penn SG, He L, Natan MJ. Nanoparticles for bioanalysis. *Curr Opin Chem Biol*. 2003 Oct;7(5):609-15.

[7] Laval JM, Mazeran PE, Thomas D. Nanobiotechnology and its role in the modern construction of modern analytical devices. *Analyst*. 2000 Jan;125(1):29-33.

[8] Patel GM, Patel GC, Patel RB, Patel JK, Patel M. Nanorobot: a versatile tool in nanomedicine. *J Drug Focus*. 2006 Feb;14(2):63-7.

[9] Baba Y. Nanotechnology in medicine. *Nippon Rinsho*. 2006 Feb;64(2):189-98.

[10] Cao R, Villalonga R, Fragoso A. Towards nanomedicine with a supramolecular approach: a review. *IEE Proc Nanobiotechnol*. 2005 Oct;152(5):159-64.

[11] Jain KK. Applications of Nanobiotechnology in Clinical Diagnostics. *Clin Chem*. 2007 Sep 21;

[12] Jain KK. Applications of biochips: from diagnostics to personalized medicine. *Curr Opin Drug Discov Devel*. 2004 May;7(3):285-9.

[13] Murthy SK. Nanoparticles in modern medicine: state of the art and future challenges. *Int J Nanomedicine*. 2007;2(2):129-41.

[14] Pauwels EK, Erba P Towards the use of nanoparticles in cancer therapy and imaging. *Drug Moderns Perspect*. 2007 May;20(4):213-20.

[15] Moghimi SM, Hunter AC, Murray JC. Nanomedicine: current status and future prospects. *FASEB J*. 2005 Mar;19(3):311-30.

[16] Emerich DF. Nanomedicine--prospective therapeutic and diagnostic applications. *Expert Opin Biol Ther*. 2005 Jan;5(1):1-5.

[17] Nakayama M, Okano T. Drug delivery systems using nano-sized drug carriers. *Gan To Kagaku Ryoho*. 2005 Jul;32(7):935-40.

[18] Erickson RP. From "magic bullet" to "specially engineered shotgun loads": the modern genetics and the need for individualized pharmacotherapy. *Bioessays*. 1998 Aug;20(8):683-5.

[19] Osieka R. Oncology. *Arzneimittelforschung*. 1997 Oct;47(10):1161-5.

[20] Galanski M, Keppler BK. Searching for the magic bullet: anticancer platinum drugs which can be accumulated or activated in the tumor tissue. *Anticancer Agents Med Chem*. 2007 Jan;7(1):55-73.

[21] Welch DR. Biologic considerations for drug focusing in cancer illed subjects. *Cancer Treat Rev*. 1987 Dec;14(3-4):351-8.

[22] Kreuter MW. Human behavior and cancer. Forget the magic bullet! *Cancer*. 1993 Aug 1;72(3 Suppl):996-1001.

[23] Couvreur P, Vauthier C. Nanotechnology: intelligent design to treat complex disease. *Pharm Res*. 2006 Jul;23(7):1417-50.

[24] Chen HC. Modern era of reconstructive microsurgery. *Changgeng Yi Xue Za Zhi*. 1997 Sep;20(3):153-62.

[25] Chicarilli ZN. Pediatric microsurgery: revascularization and replantation. *J Pediatr Surg*. 1986 Aug;21(8):706-10.

[26] Arnold DJ, Wax MK; Microvascular Committee of the American Academy of Otolaryngology--Head and Neck Surgery. Pediatric microvascular reconstruction: a report from the Microvascular Committee. *Otolaryngol Head Neck Surg*. 2007 May;136(5):848-51.

[27] Strasburger VC. First do no harm: why have parents and pediatricians missed the boat on children and media? *J Pediatr*. 2007 Oct;151(4):334-6.

[28] Smoyak SA. Primum non nocere (first, do no harm). *J Psychosoc Nurs Ment Health Serv*. 2007 Sep;45(9):8-9.

[29] Evans J. First, do no harm. *Pract Midwife*. 2007 Sep;10(8):22-3.

[30] Monreal M, Trujillo-Santos J. Emerging Way of thoughts in Clinical Practice Guidelines. *Z Gastroenterol*. 2007 Oct;45(10):1075-1081.

[31] Freitas RA Jr. Nanotechnology, nanomedicine and nanosurgery. *Int J Surg*. 2005;3(4):243-6. Epub 2005 Nov 28.

[32] Ebbesen M, Jensen TG. Nanomedicine: techniques, potentials, and ethical implications. *J Biomed Biotechnol*. 2006;2006(5):51516.

[33] Fankhauser F, Niederer PF, Kwasniewska S, van der Zypen E. Supernormal vision, high-resolution retinal imaging, multiphoton imaging and nanosurgery of the cornea--a review. *Technol Health Care*. 2004;12(6):443-53.

[34] Freitas RA Jr. Nanodentistry. *J Am Dent Assoc*. 2000 Nov;131(11):1559-65.

[35] Putnam D. Polymers for gene delivery across length scales. *Nat Mater*. 2006 Jun;5(6):439-51.

[36] Piskin E, Dincer S, Turk M. Gene delivery: intelligent but just at the beginning. *J Biomater Sci Polym Ed*. 2004;15(9):1181-202.

[37] Chowdhury EH, Akaike T. Bio-functional inorganic materials: an attractive branch of gene-based nano-medicine delivery for 21st century. *Curr Gene Ther*. 2005 Dec;5(6):669-76.

[38] Bhavsar MD, Amiji MM. Polymeric nano- and microparticle technologies for oral gene delivery. *Expert Opin Drug Deliv*. 2007 May;4(3):197-213.

[39] Chen H, Titushkin I, Stroscio M, Cho M. Altered membrane dynamics of quantum dot-conjugated integrins during osteogenic differentiation of human bone marrow derived progenitor cells. *Biophys J*. 2007 Feb 15;92(4):1399-408.

[40] Garon EB, Marcu L, Luong Q, Tcherniantchouk O, Crooks GM, Koeffler HP. Quantum dot labeling and tracking of human leukemic, bone marrow and cord blood cells. *Leuk Res*. 2007 May;31(5):643-51.

[41] Horak D, Babic M, Jendelova P, Herynek V, Trchova M, Pientka Z, Pollert E, Hajek M, Sykova E. D-mannose-modified iron oxide nanoparticles for stem cell labeling. *Bioconjug Chem*. 2007 May-Jun;18(3):635-44.

[42] Zheng J, Ghazani AA, Song Q, Mardyani S, Chan WC, Wang C. Cellular imaging and surface marker labeling of hematopoietic cells using quantum dot bioconjugates. *Lab Hematol*. 2006;12(2):94-8.

[43] West JL. "Nano-technologies for biomedical applications". *Conf Proc IEEE Eng Med Biol Soc*. 2006;1:nil19-20.

[44] Levy I, Shoseyov O. Cross bridging proteins in nature and their utilization in bio- and nanotechnology. *Curr Protein Pept Sci*. 2004 Feb;5(1):33-49.

[45] Smith LA, Ma PX. Nano-fibrous scaffolds for tissue engineering. *Colloids Surf B Biointerfaces*. 2004 Dec 10;39(3):125-31.

[46] Kikuchi A, Okano T. Nanostructured designs of biomedical materials: applications of cell sheet engineering to functional regenerative tissues and organs. *J Control Release*. 2005 Jan 3;101(1-3):69-84.

[47] Murugan R, Ramakrishna S. Nano-featured scaffolds for tissue engineering: a review of spinning methodologies. *Tissue Eng*. 2006 Mar;12(3):435-47.

[48] Staples M, Daniel K, Cima MJ, Langer R. Application of Micro- and Nano-Electromechanical Devices to Drug Delivery. *Pharm Res*. 2006 May 5;

[49] Erickson RP. From "magic bullet" to "specially engineered shotgun loads": the modern genetics and the need for individualized pharmacotherapy. *Bioessays*. 1998 Aug;20(8):683-5.

[50] Osieka R. Oncology. *Arzneimittelforschung*. 1997 Oct;47(10):1161-5.

[51] Galanski M, Keppler BK. Searching for the magic bullet: anticancer platinum drugs which can be accumulated or activated in the tumor tissue. *Anticancer Agents Med Chem*. 2007 Jan;7(1):55-73.

[52] Welch DR. Biologic considerations for drug focusing in cancer illed subjects. *Cancer Treat Rev*. 1987 Dec;14(3-4):351-8.

[53] Kreuter MW. Human behavior and cancer. Forget the magic bullet! *Cancer*. 1993 Aug 1;72(3 Suppl):996-1001.

[54] Couvreur P, Vauthier C. Nanotechnology: intelligent design to treat complex disease. *Pharm Res*. 2006 Jul;23(7):1417-50.

[55] Ullman D. Let's have a serious discussion of nanopharmacology and homeopathy. *FASEB J*. 2006 Dec;20(14):2661; author reply 2662. No

[56] Yokoyama M.Drug focusing with nano-sized carrier systems. *J Artif Organs*. 2005;8(2):77-84.

[57] Sahoo SK, Labhasetwar V. Nanotech approaches to drug delivery and imaging. *Drug Discov Today*. 2003 Dec 15;8(24):1112-20.

[58] Cachau RE, Gonzalez-Nilo FD, Ventura ON, Fritts MJ. In-silico nanobio-design. A modern frontier in computational biology. *Curr Top Med Chem*. 2007;7(15):1537-40.

[59] Loew GH, Villar HO, Alkorta I. Strategies for indirect computer-aided drug design. *Pharm Res*. 1993 Apr;10(4):475-86.

[60] Serruto, D., Rappuoli, R. Post-genomic vaccine modern construction. *FEBS Lett*. 2006; 580: 2985-92.

[61] Scarselli, M., Giuliani, M.M., Adu-Bobie, J., Pizza, M., Rappuoli, R. The impact of genomics on vaccine design. *Trends Biotechnol*. 2005; 23: 84-91.

[62] Capecchi, B., Serruto, D., Adu-Bobie, J., Rappuoli, R., Pizza, M. The genome revolution in vaccine research. *Curr Issues Mol Biol* 2004; 6: 17-27.

[63] Wiwanitkit V.

[64] Dhiman, N., Bonilla, R., O'Kane, D,J., Poland, G.A. Gene expression microarrays: a 21st century tool for directed vaccine design. *Vaccine* 2001; 20: 22-30.

[65] Grandi, G. Rational antibacterial vaccine design through genomic technologies. *Int J Parasitol*. 2003; 35: 615 - 20.

[66] 18. Barry, M.A., Howell, D.P., Andersson, H.A., Chen, J.L., Singh, R.A. Expression library immunization to discover and improve vaccine antigens. *Immunol Rev*. 2004; 199; 68 - 83.

[67] Betton, J.M. Rapid and highly efficient, the recombinational cloning technology is largely used for structural genomics and functional proteomics. *Biochimie*. 2004; 86: 601-5.

[68] Dieckman, L.J., Hanly,W.C., Collart, E.R. Strategies for high-throughput gene cloning and expression. *Genet Eng (N Y)*. 2006; 27: 179-90.

[69] Davies, D.H., Liang, X., Hernandez, J.E. et al.. Profiling the humoral immune response to infection by using proteome microarrays: high-throughput vaccine and diagnostic antigen discomuch. *Proc Natl Acad Sci U S* A. 2005; 102: 547-52.

[70] Zagursky RJ, Russell D. Bioinformatics: use in bacterial vaccine discomuch. *Biotechniques*. 2001; 31: 636, 638, 640.

[71] Schonbach, C., Nagashima, T., Konagaya, A. Textmining in support of knowledge discomuch for vaccine modern construction. *Methods*. 2004; 34: 488-95.

[72] Flower, D.R., McSparron, H., Blythe, M.J. et al.. Computational vaccinology: quantitative approaches. *Novartis Found Symp*. 2003; 254: 102-20.

[73] Brusic, V., August, J.T., Petrovsky, N. Information technologies for vaccine research. *Expert Rev Vaccines*. 2005; 4: 407-17.

[74] Schuster D, Steindl TM, Langer T. Predicting drug metabolism induction in silico. *Curr Top Med Chem*. 2006;6(15):1627-40.

[75] Ekins S, Mestres J, Testa B. In silico pharmacology for drug discomuch: applications to focus and beyond. *Br J Pharmacol*. 2007 Sep;152(1):21-37.

[76] Rollinger JM, Langer T, Stuppner H. Integrated in silico tools for exploiting the natural products' bioactivity. *Planta Med*. 2006 Jun;72(8):671-8.

[77] Thibaut U. Bioinformatics and rational drug design: tools for discomuch and better understanding of biological focus and mode of action of drugs. *Scand J Gastroenterol Suppl*. 2002;(236):95-9.

[78] Hirono S. An introduction to the computer-aided structure-based drug design--applications of bioinformatics to drug discomuch. *Rinsho Byori*. 2002 Jan;50(1):45-51.

[79] Fischer HP. Towards quantitative biology: integration of biological information to elucidate disease pathways and to guide drug discomuch. *Biotechnol Annu Rev*. 2005;11:1-68.

[80] Jain KK. Challenges of drug discomuch for personalized medicine. *Curr Opin Mol Ther*. 2006 Dec;8(6):487-92.

[81] Morrow KJ Jr, Bawa R, Wei C. Recent advances in basic and clinical nanomedicine. *Med Clin North Am*. 2007 Sep;91(5):805-43.

[82] Nie S, Xing Y, Kim GJ, Simons JW. PharmaMedDevice 2007. Issues in nanodrug delivery and personalized medicine. *IDrugs*. 2007 Jul;10(7):455-8.

[83] Baba Y. Nanotechnology in medicine. *Nippon Rinsho*. 2006 Feb;64(2):189-98.

[84] Tsai CJ, Zheng J, Aleman C, Nussinov R. Structure by design: from single proteins and their building blocks to nanostructures. *Trends Biotechnol*. 2006 Oct;24(10):449-54.

[85] Wei C, Wei W, Morris M, Kondo E, Gorbounov M, Tomalia DA. Nanomedicine and drug delivery. *Med Clin North Am*. 2007 Sep;91(5):863-70.

[86] Conti M, Tazzari V, Baccini C, Pertici G, Serino LP, De Giorgi U. Anticancer drug delivery with nanoparticles. *In Vivo*. 2006 Nov-Dec;20(6A):697-701.

[87] Liu Y, Miyoshi H, Nakamura M. Nanomedicine for drug delivery and imaging: a promising avenue for cancer therapy and diagnosis using focused functional nanoparticles. *Int J Cancer*. 2007 Jun 15;120(12):2527-37.

[88] Shaffer C. Nanomedicine transforms drug delivery. *Drug Discov Today*. 2005 Dec;10(23-24):1581-2.

[89] Kim KY. Nanotechnology platforms and physiological challenges for cancer therapeutics. *Nanomedicine*. 2007 Jun;3(2):103-10.

[90] Rotomskis R, Streckyte G, Karabanovas V. Nanoparticles in diagnostics and therapy: towards nanomedicine. *Medicina (Kaunas)*. 2006;42(7):542-58.

[91] Ashammakhi N. Nanosize, mega-impact, potential for medical applications of nanotechnology. *J Craniofac Surg*. 2006 Jan;17(1):3-7.

[92] Ravi Kumar MN. Nano and microparticles as controlled drug delivery devices. *J Pharm Pharm Sci*. 2000 May-Aug;3(2):234-58.

[93] Pizzi M, De Martiis O, Grasso V. Fabrication of self assembled micro reservoirs for controlled drug release. *Biomed Microdevices*. 2004 Jun;6(2):155-8.

[94] Zhou JJ, Chen RF, Tang QB, Zhou QB, Lu HW, Wang J. Preparation of 5-fluorouracil encapsulated in amphiphilic polysaccharide nano-micelles and its killing effect on hepatocarcinoma cell line HepG2. *Ai Zheng*. 2006 Dec;25(12):1459-63.

[95] Pattani AS, Mandawgade SD, Patravale VB. Modern construction and comparative anti-microbial evaluation of lipid nanoparticles and nanoemulsion of Polymyxin B. *J Nanosci Nanotechn*ol. 2006 Sep-Oct;6(9-10):2986-90.

[96] Liu J, Zeng F, Allen C. In vivo fate of unimers and micelles of a poly(ethylene glycol)-block-poly(caprolactone) copolymer in mice following intravenous administration. *Eur J Pharm Biopharm*. 2007 Mar;65(3):309-19.

[97] Liu J, Zeng F, Allen C. In vivo fate of unimers and micelles of a poly(ethylene glycol)-block-poly(caprolactone) copolymer in mice following intravenous administration. *Eur J Pharm Biopharm*. 2007 Mar;65(3):309-19.

[98] Cevc G. Lipid vesicles and other colloids as drug carriers on the skin. *Adv Drug Deliv Rev*. 2004 Mar 27;56(5):675-711.

[99] Fang JY. Nano- or submicron-sized liposomes as carriers for drug delivery. *Chang Gung Med J*. 2006 Jul-Aug;29(4):358-62.

[100] Allen TM, Cheng WW, Hare JI, Laginha KM. Pharmacokinetics and pharmacodynamics of lipidic nano-particles in cancer. *Anticancer Agents Med Chem*. 2006 Nov;6(6):513-23.

[101] Vonarbourg A, Passirani C, Saulnier P, Benoit JP. Parameters influencing the stealthiness of colloidal drug delivery systems. *Biomaterials*. 2006 Aug;27(24):4356-73.

[102] Yokoyama M, Okano T. Focusing of anti-cancer drugs with nano-sized carrier system. *Nippon Rinsho*. 1998 Dec;56(12):3227-34.

[103] Ariga K, Hill JP, Ji Q. Layer-by-layer assembly as a versatile bottom-up nanofabrication technique for exploratory research and realistic application. *Phys Chem Chem Phys*. 2007 May 21;9(19):2319-40.

[104] Nimjee SM, Rusconi CP, Sullenger BA. Aptamers: an emerging class of therapeutics. *Annu Rev Med*. 2005;56:555-83.

[105] Oku N, Namba Y. Long-circulating liposomes. *Crit Rev Ther Drug Carrier Syst*. 1994;11(4):231-70.

[106] Oku N. Basic study and application of functional liposomes. *Yakugaku Zasshi*. 1995 Jul;115(7):483-98.

[107] Meers P. Enzyme-activated focusing of liposomes. *Adv Drug Deliv Rev*. 2001 Dec 31;53(3):265-72.

[108] Bai S, Thomas C, Rawat A, Ahsan F. Recent progress in dendrimer-based nanocarriers. *Crit Rev Ther Drug Carrier Syst*. 2006;23(6):437-95.

[109] Benson HA. Transfersomes for transdermal drug delivery. *Expert Opin Drug Deliv.* 2006 Nov;3(6):727-37.

[110] Lee LA, Wang Q. Adaptations of nanoscale viruses and other protein cages for medical applications. *Nanomedicine.* 2006 Sep;2(3):137-49.

[111] Corradin G. Antigen processing and presentation. *Immunol Lett.* 1990 Aug;25(1-3):11-3.

[112] Bijker MS, Melief CJ, Offringa R, van der Burg SH. Design and modern construction of synthetic peptide vaccines: past, present and future. *Expert Rev Vaccines.* 2007 Aug;6(4):591-603.

[113] Sette A, Peters B. Immune epitope mapping in the post-genomic era: lessons for vaccine modern construction. *Curr Opin Immunol.* 2007 Feb;19(1):106-10.

[114] Ontology annotation: mapping genomic parts to biological function. *Curr Opin Chem* Biol. 2007 Feb;11(1):4-11.

[115] Marchant GE, Sylvester DJ. Transnational models for regulation of nanotechnology. *J Law Med Ethics.* 2006 Winter;34(4):714-25.

[116] Wiwanitkit V. Ethics of clinical pathologist. *J Med Assoc Thai.* 2006 Dec;89(12):2161-2.

[117] Resnik DB, Tinkle SS. Ethics in nanomedicine. *Nanomed.* 2007 Jun;2(3):345-50.

[118] Khushf G. Systems theory and the ethics of human enhancement: a framework for NBIC convergence. *Ann N Y Acad Sci.* 2004 May;1013:124-49.

[119] Sententia W. Neuroethical considerations: cognitive liberty and converging technologies for improving human cognition. *Ann N Y Acad Sci.* 2004 May;1013:221-8.

[120] Grunwald A. Nanotechnology--a new field of ethical inquiry? *Sci Eng Ethics.* 2005 Apr;11(2):187-201.

Chapter III

QUANTUM THERAPY AS WELL AS PHOTON THERAPY

WHAT IS "QUANTUM"?

Quantum is a physical term that implies the smallest discrete amount of some physical property that a system can have. Quantum theory, the branch of physics which is based on quantization, started in 1900 when Planck published his theory explaining the emission spectrum of black bodies [1-3]. The bippoasesic of radiation as well as matter is the heart of the quantum theory. In physics, quantum mechanics is the learning of the relationship between energy or radiation as well as matter, in particular that between valence shell electrons as well as photons. Bohr's theory is the root for the generation of the present quantum physics [4-5]. Bohr's atomic theory is broadly viewed as remarkable, both for its accuracy in predicting the observed optical transitions of one-electron atoms as well as for its failure to fully correspond with current electronic structure theory [6]. However, what is not routinely appreciated is that Bohr's classical semiclassical conception differed significantly from the Bohr-Sommerfeld theory as well as offers an alternative semiclassical approximation scheme with remarkable attributes [6]. It is routinely believed that the old quantum theory, as presented by Bohr in 1913, fails when adapted to few electron systems, such as the H(2) molecule [7]. Bohr's classical method did not impose action quantization constraints but rather obtained these as predictions by simply matching photon as well as classical orbital frequencies [6]. The discovery of the efficacy-quantum by Planck as well as further work of Borh was the fundamental contributing root to Einstein's hypothesis of lightquanta [8]. With the mentioned fundamental theories, Einstein could explain the external light-electrical effect [8]. The work of Einstein is the root of the modern ppoasese of science. As a case study, there was a long track from the concept of stimulated emission as the fundamental idea of laser technical work by Albert Einstein in 1917 to the practical use of the laser ar present [9]. It is also the fundamental for the modern science, quantum mechanics. Quantum mechanics is a fundamental branch of physics with wide applications in both experimental as well as theoretical physics [10-13]. The quantum theory is the theoretical basis of modern physics that can be valuable in explaining the nature as well as behavior of matter as well as energy on the atomic as well as subatomic level. Conrad said that biological cells had greater information processing efficiency than the programmable computers used to model them [12]. Conrad also suggested that systems in which quantum features played a prominent work are more powerful than classical physical-dynamical analogs [12].

Quantum medicine is the modern kind of medicine. Naturally, all things, chemicals, plants, animals as well as human beings are composed of various tissues, organs, cells, molecules, as well as atoms. The combinations of atoms lead to molecules. The combinations of molecules lead to cells. The combinations of cells results in tissues. The combinations of tissues lead to organs. The combinations of organs lead to human beings. Fundamentally, an atom consists of electron as well as nuclei which intern quantum as well as neutron. Electron poses negative charge, proton poses positive charge as well as neutron poses neutral charge. Normally human beings cannot see the atom. In addition, the compositions of atom are beyond human reach. But according to the modern elementary particle theory, elementary particle is considered to have immense size as well as types, as well as it poases property as energy field which rotates as well as vibrates itself. With the advent in nanoscience, those very tiny compositions can be studied.

Quantum determination method is the determination technique, which tests the energy composed of magnetic energy generated by quantum as well as electron movement. Improvements in quantum chemical techniques have led to increased applications to biological problems, including the generation of potential energy functions for molecular mechanics as well as modeling of the reactive chemistry in enzyme active sites, with particularly interesting progress being constructed for metal-containing systems [13]. The three items to be considered in quantum determination method are (a) use of quantum mechanical electronic structure techniques such as molecular orbital theory as well as density functional theory, usually in conjunction with molecular mechanics; (b) treating vibrational motions quantum mechanically, either in an instantaneous harmonic approximation, or by path integrals, or by a three-dimensional wave function coupled to classical nuclear motion; (c) incorporation of multidimensional tunneling approximations into reaction rate calculations [14]. Orbital theory is the fundamental knowledge for quantum chemistry. Molecular orbital analytical work is the fundamental technique for study of quantum mechanical electronic structure. To assist molecular orbital analytical work, there are several modern computation instruments for performing this analytical aim. As a case study, AOMix is a modern user-friendly software for the molecular orbital analytical work [15]. It calculates the molecular orbital compositions in terms of the constituent chemical parts in the molecule or atom [15]. AOMix automatically processes output files of multiple quantum-chemical packages [15]. AOMix also permits to deeply review chemical structure making use of overlap populations (total as well as per molecular orbital), valence indices, 2-center (Mayer, Lowdin, Wiberg, as well as bond-order symmetry components) as well as 3- as well as 4-center bond orders, charge decomposition orbital, CDA (total, per molecular orbital, per symmetry type), as well as condensed Fukui functions [15]. Conventional quantum chemistry techniques are either too expensive to apply to large systems or too approximate for the results to be reliable, as well as they fail to satisfy this requirement [16]. A variety of different approaches is being developed with the aim of achieving this goal: local correlation techniques; divide-as well as-conquer techniques; linear-scaling density functional techniques based on the fast multiple as well as other approximations; effective potential techniques; as well as hybrid techniques [16].

The influence as well as application of quantum determination on medical field is named "quantum medicine". Quantum medicine is one of the most promising tracks of modern contemporary medicine [17-18]. It is based on the use of aimful effects of low-dosage electromagnetic radiation or quantum in treatment, diagnosis, prophylaxis, as well as rehabilitation of patients.

Quantum Diagnosis: Stage Before Treatment

Application of quantum medicine diagnosis is a main focus. This is far away from basic nanodiagnosis. Indeed, the genesis of nanotechnology leads to the promise of revolutionary advances across medicine, communications, genomics and robotics [1]. Nanodiagnosis is a diagnostic technique using nanoparticle. Nanomaterials and nanotechnology combined with modern instrumentation have the potential to address this emerging technology. Using a variety of nanomaterials for multiplex diagnostics and imaging applications will lead to sensitive, rapid and cost-effective solutions for the modern clinical laboratory. Nanowire and nanoporous approaches into genomics and proteomics could help increase the sensitivity and accuracy of diagnostics and would shorten the time of diagnostic procedures that will further improve the efficiency of medical treatment. Basically, different nanomaterials can be applied for medical diagnostic usage. Among the different nanomaterials used to generate nanoparticles, are organic polymers, co-polymers and metals. Some of these materials can self assemble, and depending on the conditions under which the self-assembly process occurs, a vast array of shapes can be generated. Quantum diagnosis is the next generation of simple nanodiagnosis.

There are several attempts to develop a modern diagnostic instrument at quantum level [19-20]. Quantum diagnosis relies on energy as well as information parameters that specifically as well as depicts both the general state of the organism as well as its organs, systems as well as interrelations. Determinations of relevant electric parameters at certain points of the body surface permit to diagnose for a disease or to identify it at the early onset stage with high accuracy. Determinations of those parameters are also assistable to define predisposition of the patient to specific disease. In nanomedicine, a well-known diagnostic instrument namely quantum dot is now available. Quantum dot is a synthesized nanopolymer with semiconductor property. Quantum dot is a novel class of inorganic fluorophore which are gaining widespread interest as a result of their exceptional photophysical properties. Semiconductor quantum dots are inorganic nanoparticles with unique photophysical properties [21]. In particular, their huge one- as well as two-photon absorption cross sections, tunable emission bas well ass as well as excellent photobleaching resistances are stimulating the generation of luminescent probes for biomedical imaging as well as sensing applications [21]. With the nanoproperty of quantum dot, electron as well as energy transfer processes can be designed to interprete the luminescence of semiconductor quantum dots in response to molecular recognition events [21]. On the basis of these operating principles, the presence of target analytes can be transduced into detectable luminescence signals. Quantum dot is broadly applicable for staining of living cells. The quantum dot is more stable than classical fluorescence staining, which was accepted as one of the most promising cas well asidates for chemical sensing [22]. At present, squantum dots have been increasingly employed in measuring the dynamic behavior of biomacromolecules making use of fluorescence correlation spectroscopy [23]. This leads to a challenge, because quantum dots display their own dynamic behavior in the form of intermittent photoluminescence, also known as blinking [23].

Bioconjugated nanoparticles as well as quantum dots are among the most exciting nanomaterials with promising application potentials in nanomedicine field [24]. Although most of these applications are based on the optical properties of nanoparticle materials such as surface plasmon resonance, surface enhanced Raman scattering as well as strong photoluminescence, other items of nanoparticles such as the catalytic effect as well as amplification effect associated with the nanoscale dimension have also been explored [24]. In addition to stas well asard quantum dot, now functional antibodies, antibodies that are sterically available for functional binding to target proteins can be successfully conjugated to semiconductor quantum dots [25]. This is a modern potential strategy for improving quantum dot labeling of biological preparations [25]. However, Pathak et al. found that the number of available functional antibodies varied significantly for different conjugation techniques as well as were lower than previously estimated [26]. Pathak et al. said that these results might suggest potential strategies for improving quantum dot labeling of biological preparations [26].

In addition to antibody, conjugation can be constructed use of other substances. Another broadly used substance is peptide. In 2005, Tomlinson et al. prepared peptide-quantum dot conjugates by attaching angiotensin II (Ang II) to cadmium selenide/zinc sulfide core-shell nanocrystals making use of an 1-[3-(Dimethyamino)propyl]-3-ethylcarbo diimide hydrochloride (EDC) coupling [27]. According to this work, the Ang II-quantum dot conjugates did not bind to parental cells as well as showed similar staining patterns when compared with a commercially available conjugate [27]. Young as well as Rozengurt demonstrated that quantum dot-ANG II was brighter as well as more photostable than agonist labeled with the organic dye Cy3 [28]. Young as well as Rozengurt demonstrated that quantum dot technical work could be adapted to monitor ligas well as binding to G protein-coupled receptors [28]. In 2007, Tsay et al. reported the study on singlet oxygen production by peptide-coated quantum dot-photosensitizer conjugates [29]. Tsay et al. found that the conjugate could be simultaneously used for fluorescence imaging as well as singlet oxygen generation [29]. In addition, singlet oxygen quantum yields as high as 0.31 were achieved making use of 532-nm excitation wavelengths [29].

Quantum dot can also be adapted for imaging [30]. The modern generations of quantum dots have far-reaching potential for the study of intracellular processes at the single-molecule level, high-resolution cellular imaging, long-term in vivo observation of cell trafficking, tumor targeting, as well as diagnostics [31]. Quantum dots are emerging as a superior alternative as well as are poised to change the world of bio-imaging as well as further its applications in fundamental as well as adapted biology [31-35]. Jaiswal as well as Simon said that the improved synthesis of water-stable quantum dots, the generation of approaches to label cells efficiently with quantum dots, as well as improvements in conjugating quantum dots to specific biological molecules had triggered the recent explosion in their use in biological imaging [36]. Jaiswal as well as Simon also noted that although there had been several successes in making use of quantum dots for biological applications, limitations remained that required solution before these powerful instruments could be used routinely by biologists [36].

QUANTUM TREATMENT

Quantum treatment is a treatment based on quantum [37-38]. Quantum treatment recruits natural, environment like factors of electromagnetic exposure that poases beneficial effects on cells, organs as well as system of the organism. It is accepted that low level of energy used in quantum medicine is absolutely harmless. The treatment reserves existing anomalous process, disease, to stability as well as health. This is because quantum treatment activates latent reserves of the organism adaptation both at the cellular level as well as whole biologic system, strongly enhancing immunity as well as mobilizing the organism for active resistance to functional disorder. Quantum medicine is increasingly adapted in treatment for all fields of medicine. It is broadly used in cases of cancer, radiation sickness, cardiovascular diseases, locomotors diseases, infantile cerebral palsy, urolithiasis, bronchial asthma, alopecia, enuresis as well as infertility. Optical quantum generators or laser is the best example of quantum treatment. The optical quantum generators are valuable in orthopedics/ traumatology, genecology, urology, sports medicine, dermatology, dentistry, surgery, neurology as well as rheumatology [39-45]. Indeed, the quantum therapy poases a long history. The classical well-known therapy is the phototherapy in infantile hyperbilirubinemia [46]. In phototherapy, the structural photoisomerization is routinely assumed to represent the main route of bilirubin elimination [47]. As a consequence, the determination of the spectral bas well as that optimizes the process of formation of lumirubin in neonate may represent an important step in the improvement of the clinical protocol of phototherapy [47]. The laser therapy is another classical treatment as previously mentioned. Not only the treatment by the classical quantum medical instrument. The drug treatment for general diseases also base on the principle of quantum change.

Based on advent of nanobiotechnical work, quantum dot can also be adapted for quantum treatment. At present, the photophysics of singlet oxygen generation in relation to quantum dot-based energy transfer is broadly discussed as well as the possibility of making use of quantum dots as photosensitizer in photodynamic therapy is broadly assessed, including their current limitations to applications in biological systems [48-49]. Fundamentally, photodynamic therapy is an emerging treatment modality for a range of disease classes, both cancerous as well as noncancerous [51]. This work brought about an active pursuit of modern photodynamic therapy agents that can be optimized for the unique set of photophysical characteristics that are required for a successful clinical agent [50-51]. Hsieh et al. reported the success in design as well as synthesis of Ir-complex functionalized CdSe/ZnS quantum dots, in which the QD played a key work in imaging, while the Ir-complex acted as a sensitizer to produce singlet oxygen for photodynamic therapy aim [52].

Table 1. Important reports on photon therapy

Authors	Details
Nadig et al. [57]	Nadig et al. reported on usefulness of 99mTc-pertechnetate single-photon emission computed tomography in remnant mass estimation of postsurgical patients of differentiated thyroid cancer during internal dosimetry [57].
Boogers et al. [58]	Boogers et al. reported on myocardial perfusion single photon emission computed tomography for the assessment of mechanical dyssynchrony [58].
Trimble et al. [59]	Trimble et al. reported on the role of myocardial perfusion imaging to evaluate patients for cardiac resynchronization therapy [59].
Nguyen et al. [60]	Nguyen et al. reported on proton-beam versus intensity-modulated radiation therapy for treatment of prostate cancer [60]. Nguyen et al. concluded that supported the use of protons in prostate cancer [60]
Suit et al. [61]	Suit et al. proposed that the rationale for the proposals that prior to a wider use of proton radiation therapy should be supported by data from phase III clinical trials [61]. Suit et al. concluded that proton therapy provided superior distributions of low LET radiation dose relative to that by photon therapy for treatment of a large proportion of tumor or normal tissue situations [61].
Schneider et al. [62]	Schneider et al. reported on effect of proton radiotherapy on secondary cancer incidence [62]. They concluded that 6-MV photons provided only a moderate risk [62].
Konski et al. [63]	Konski et al. studied if proton beam therapy was cost effective in the treatment of adenocarcinoma of the prostate [63]. Konski et al. concluded that proton beam therapy was not cost effective for most patients with prostate cancer [63].
Mock et al. [64]	Mock et al. studied on comparative treatment planning on localized prostate carcinoma conformal photon- versus proton-based radiotherapy [64]. According to this work, Mock et al. concluded that the advantageous dose distribution of proton-beam therapy for prostate cancer might result in decreased side effects, which needs to be confirmed in clinical studies [64].
Weber et al. [65]	Weber et al. reported that reducing the size of the proton pencil beam by using the mini-beam mode improved the dose homogeneity, but this did not have a significant effect on the dose conformity [65].
DeLaney [66}	DeLaney reported that proton radiation therapy brought several potential treatment advantages to patients that could be studied in the setting of clinical trials and the patients' willingness to enter these clinical trials was also quite high [66].
Fontenot et al. [67]	Fontenot et al. reported that proton therapy decreased the integral therapeutic dose required for local control in prostate patients compared to intensity-modulated radiotherapy [67].
Cella et al. [68]	Cella et al. performed a study to assess the potential benefit of intensity modulated proton beams in optimizing the dose distribution to safely escalate the tumor dose in prostate cancer radiotherapy [68]. Cella et al. concluded that proton therapy could be an interesting alternative [68].
Weber et al. [69]	Weber et al. reported on the possibility of using radiation therapy planning with photons and protons for early and advanced breast cancer [69].
Goitein and Jermann [70]	Goitein and Jermann studied on the relative costs of proton and X-ray radiation therapy [70]. Goitein and Jermann concluded that proton beam therapy was clinically worthwhile is a cost-effectiveness track [70].
Paganetti et al. [71]	Paganetti et al. reported on relative biological effectiveness (RBE) values for proton beam therapy [71]. Paganetti et al. concluded that there was a clear requirement for prospective assessments of normal tissue reactions in proton irradiated patients and [71].
Weber et al. [72]	Weber et al. found that the use of linear accelerator-based stereotactic radiotherapy photon techniques, compared with protons, can result in similar levels of dose conformation [72].

In addition to therapy, quantum prophylaxis can also be performed based on the techniques of quantum therapy. For instance, prophylaxis of disease relapses in periodical exacerbation requires quantum treatment at early stage of an epidemic. There are also some interesting reports on application of quantum dot in vaccinology. Upadhyay investigated how mild local hyperthermia could be used for transdermal-immunization [53]. Upadhyay said that hyperthermia enhanced transdermal-immunization procedure was likely to have higher compliance as it did not cause any pain or visible damage to the skin [53]. Quantum rehabilitation also makes use of quantum therapy techniques. The use of quantum medicine technologies can assist fasten patient rehabilitation period after complex operations, radiation nor chemical exposures. The most broadly use quantum rehabilitation is for cardiological problem [54-55]. The quantum gravitational therapy is the broadly mentioned method. This technique is a complex therapy of myocarditis of rheumatic as well as non-rheumatic genesis making use of intravascular laser irradiation of blood, quercitrol, as well as enterosgel poases an antiinflammatory, antioxidant action, improves myocardial contractility, endowed with an antiaggregatory activity [54]. This technique is confirmed for its effectiveness in rehabilitation in myositis.his technique is confirmed for its effectiveness in rehabilitation in myositis. Nevertheless, Hossu as well as Rupert said that biophoton emission was a quantum event presented by a relatively stable but ultralow- rate emission of visible photons from living organisms as well as it poases been associated with high energy processes such as cell metabolism, growth, phagocytosis, neural activity, as well as oxidative stressive attack [56]. Hossu as well as Rupert concluded that biophoton intensity was a noninvasive indicator of the health of the human body as well as is significantly altered in different tracks by chiropractic interventions [56].

Photon Therapy

By definition, photon therapy is the treatment based on photon. The photon or positive electron is a focused interest in this modern kind of treatment. This is also strongly related to quantum therapy. However, most classical applications are used for diagnosis. New generation moves to the test for cancer treatment. Mainly focused cancerous tumor is prostate cancer in males. The details of important reports on photon therapy will be presented in Table 1.

References

[1] Shampo MA, Kyle RA. Max Planck. *JAMA*. 1980 Nov 28;244(21):2429.

[2] Cardinale AE. An adventure of the human intellect. Max Planck as well as the centenary of quantum theory. *Radiol Med (Torino)*. 2000 Mar;99(3):127-34.

[3] Staley R. On the co-creation of classical as well as modern physics. *Isis*. 2005 Dec;96(4):530-58.

[4] Shampo MA, Kyle RA. Niels Bohr. *JAMA*. 1975 Sep 1;233(9):992.

[5] del Regato JA. Niels Bohr. *Int J Radiat Oncol Biol Phys*. 1981 Apr;7(4):509-30.

[6] Svidzinsky AA, Scully MO, Herschbach DR. Bohr's 1913 molecular model revisited. *Proc Natl Acad Sci U S A*. 2005 Aug 23;102(34):11985-8.

[7] Ben-Amotz D. Revisiting Bohr's semiclassical quantum theory. *J Phys Chem B*. 2006 Oct 12;110(40):19861-6.

[8] Wiederkehr KH. Photoeffects, Einstein's light quanta as well as the history of their acceptance. *Sudhoffs Arch*. 2006;90(2):132-42.

[9] Graudenz K, Raulin C. From Einstein's Quantum Theory to modern laser therapy. The history of lasers in dermatology as well as aesthetic medicine] *Hautarzt*. 2003 Jul;54(7):575-82.

[10] Fischer-Hjalmars I. Molecular quantum mechanics in biology. *Q Rev Biophys*. 1969 Jan;1(4):311-45.

[11] Burden SJ, McKay RD. Quantum mechanics of synapses. *Cell*. 1990 Oct 5;63(1):7-8.

[12] Conrad M. Quantum mechanics as well as cellular information processing: the self-assembly paradigm. *Biomed Biochim Acta*. 1990;49(8-9):743-55.

[13] Friesner RA, Beachy MD. Quantum mechanical calculations on biological systems. *Curr Opin Struct Biol*. 1998 Apr;8(2):257-62.

[14] Gao J, Truhlar DG. Quantum mechanical techniques for enzyme kinetics. *Annu Rev Phys Chem*. 2002;53:467-505.

[15] Gorelsky SI, Lever ABP. Electronic structure as well as spectra of ruthenium diimine complexes by density functional Tteory as well as INDO/S. comparison of the two Techniques. *J Organomet Chem*. 2001; 635: 187-196.

[16] Morokuma K. Modern challenges in quantum chemistry: Quests for accurate calculations for large molecular systems. *Philos Transact A Math Phys Eng Sci*. 2002 Jun 15;360(1795):1149-64.

[17] Poases well asoll N. Energy medicine: an osteopath's personal view. *J Altern Complement Med*. 2004 Feb;10(1):87-9.

[18] Hankey A. Are we close to a theory of energy medicine? *J Altern Complement Med*. 2004 Feb;10(1):83-6.

[19] Jain KK. Applications of Nanobiotechnical work in Clinical Diagnostics. *Clin Chem*. 2007 Sep 21;

[20] Hild WA, Breunig M, Goepferich A. Quantum dots -. Nano-sized probes for the exploration of cellular as well as intracellular targeting. *Eur J Pharm Biopharm*. 2007 Jun 15;

[21] Raymo FM, Yildiz I. Luminescent chemosensors based on semiconductor quantum dots. *Phys Chem Chem Phys*. 2007 May 7;9(17):2036-43.

[22] Basabe-Desmonts L, Reinhoudt DN, Crego-Calama M. Design of fluorescent materials for chemical sensing. *Chem Soc Rev*. 2007 Jun;36(6):993-1017.

[23] Heuff RF, Swift JL, Cramb DT. Fluorescence correlation spectroscopy making use of quantum dots: advances, challenges as well as opportunities. *Phys Chem Chem Phys*. 2007 Apr 28;9(16):1870-80.

[24] Pathak S, Davidson MC, Silva GA. Characterization of the functional binding properties of antibody conjugated quantum dots. *Nano Lett*. 2007 Jul;7(7):1839-45.

[25] Huo Q. A perspective on bioconjugated nanoparticles as well as quantum dots. *Colloids Surf B Biointerfaces*. 2007 Sep 1;59(1):1-10.

[26] Pathak S, Davidson MC, Silva GA. Characterization of the functional binding properties of antibody conjugated quantum dots. *Nano Lett.* 2007 Jul;7(7):1839-45.

[27] Tomlinson ID, Mason JN, Blakely RD, Rosenthal SJ. Peptide-conjugated quantum dots: imaging the angiotensin type 1 receptor in living cells. *Techniques Mol Biol.* 2005;303:51-60.

[28] Young SH, Rozengurt E. Qdot nanocrystal conjugates conjugated to bombesin or ANG II label the cognate G protein-coupled receptor in living cells. *Am J Physiol Cell Physiol.* 2006 Mar;290(3):C728-32.

[29] Tsay JM, Trzoss M, Shi L, Kong X, Selke M, Jung ME, Weiss S. Singlet oxygen production by Peptide-coated quantum dot-photosensitizer conjugates. *J Am Chem Soc.* 2007 May 30;129(21):6865-71.

[30] Medintz IL, Uyeda HT, Goldman ER, Mattoussi H. Quantum dot bioconjugates for imaging, labelling as well as sensing. *Nat Mater.* 2005 Jun;4(6):435-46.

[31] Michalet X, Pinaud FF, Bentolila LA, Tsay JM, Doose S, Li JJ, Sundaresan G, Wu AM, Gambhir SS, Weiss S. Quantum dots for live cells, in vivo imaging, as well as diagnostics. *Science.* 2005 Jan 28;307(5709):538-44.

[32] Arya H, Kaul Z, Wadhwa R, Taira K, Hirano T, Kaul SC. Quantum dots in bio-imaging: Revolution by the small. *Biochem Biophys Res Commun.* 2005 Apr 22;329(4):1173-7.

[33] Lidke DS, Arndt-Jovin DJ. Imaging takes a quantum leap. *Physiology (Bethesda).* 2004 Dec;19:322-5.

[34] Smith AM, Nie S. Semiconductor quantum dots as biological imaging agents. *Angew Chem Int Ed Engl.* 2004 Aug 13;43(32):4129-31.

[35] Jiang W, Papa E, Fischer H, Mardyani S, Chan WC. Semiconductor quantum dots as contrast agents for whole animal imaging. *Trends Biotechnol.* 2004 Dec;22(12):607-9.

[36] Jaiswal JK, Simon SM. Potentials as well as pitfalls of fluorescent quantum dots for biological imaging. *Trends Cell Biol.* 2004 Sep;14(9):497-504.

[37] Kawasaki ES, Player A. Nanotechnical work, nanomedicine, as well as the generation of modern, effective therapies for cancer. *Nanomedicine.* 2005 Jun;1(2):101-9.

[38] Joyner JC, Purcell WP. Quantum pharmacology as well as quantitative structure-activity relationships: a brief review. *Experientia Suppl.* 1976;23:13-23.

[39] Khromov BM. Use of the optical quantum generators (lasers) in neurosurgery (literature survey). *Vopr Neirokhir.* 1974 Nov-Dec;00(6):50-3

[40] Khromov BM. Use of the optic quantum generators (lasers) in therapeutic medicine. *Klin Med (Mosk).* 1974 Nov;52(11):9-14.

[41] Khromov BM. Use of the optic quantum generators (lasers) in otorhinolaryngology. *Vestn Otorinolaringol.* 1974 Jan-Feb;(1):94-7.

[42] Moskalik KG, Kozlov AP, Akimov AA. Use of optical quantum generators (lasers) in oncology. *Vopr Onkol.* 1972;18(8):97-105.

[43] Khromov BM, Frygin NV. The use of optic quantum generators (lasers) in dermatology (a review of foreign literature). *Vestn Dermatol Venerol.* 1969 Apr;43(4):14-21.

[44] Bogdanovich UIa, Karimov MG. Use of optical quantum generators (lasers) to treat orthopedo-traumatologic patients. *Ortop Travmatol Protez*. 1984 Oct;(10):60-5.

[45] Karas well asashov VI, Petukhov EB. Quantum hemotherapy (history of the generation of the method, its mechanism of action as well as prospects for its use in dentistry). *Stomatologiia (Mosk)*. 1985 Jan-Feb;64(1):84-6.

[46] Moan J. Light therapy of modernborns with hyperbilirubinemia. *Tidsskr Nor Laegeforen*. 1992 Apr 30;112(11):1459-63.

[47] Pratesi R, Agati G, Fusi F. Phototherapy for neonatal hyperbilirubinemia. *Photodermatol*. 1989 Dec;6(6):244-57.

[48] Samia AC, Dayal S, Burda C. Quantum dot-based energy transfer: perspectives as well as potential for applications in photodynamic therapy. *Photochem Photobiol*. 2006 May-Jun;82(3):617-25.

[49] Samia AC, Chen X, Burda C. Semiconductor quantum dots for photodynamic therapy. *J Am Chem Soc*. 2003 Dec 24;125(51):15736-7.

[50] Gorman A, Killoran J, O'Shea C, Kenna T, Gallagher WM, O'Shea DF. In vitro demonstration of the heavy-atom effect for photodynamic therapy. *J Am Chem Soc*. 2004 Sep 1;126(34):10619-31.

[51] Schneider R, Tiras well as L, Frochot C, Vas well aseresse R, Thomas N, Gravier J, Guillemin F, Barberi-Heyob M. Recent improvements in the use of synthetic peptides for a selective photodynamic therapy. *Anticancer Agents Med Chem*. 2006 Sep;6(5):469-88.

[52] Hsieh JM, Ho ML, Wu PW, Chou PT, Tsai TT, Chi Y. Iridium-complex modified CdSe/ZnS quantum dots; a conceptual design for bi-functionality toward imaging as well as photosensitization. *Chem Commun (Camb)*. 2006 Feb 14;(6):615-7.

[53] Upadhyay P. Enhanced transdermal-immunization with diptheria-toxoid making use of local hyperthermia. *Vaccine*. 2006 Jul 7;24(27-28):5593-8.

[54] Ovcharova AP. The quantum gravitational therapy of myocarditis. *Lik Sprava*. 1999 Apr-May;(3):95-7.

[55] Kosov VA, Khuziev BG, Shchegol'kov AM, Nagatkin AN, Grubal'skaia IG. Spectral quantum therapy as a part of resort's rehabilitation program for patients with myocardial infarction. *Vopr Kurortol Fizioter Lech Fiz Kult*. 2001 Jul-Aug;(4):9-13.

[56] Hossu M, Rupert R. Quantum events of biophoton emission associated with complementary as well as alternative medicine therapies: a descriptive pilot study. *J Altern Complement Med*. 2006 Mar;12(2):119-24.

[57] Nadig MR, Pant GS, Bal C. Usefulness of 99mTc-pertechnetate single-photon emission computed tomography in remnant mass estimation of postsurgical patients of differentiated thyroid cancer during internal dosimetry. *Nucl Med Commun*. 2008 Sep;29(9):809-14.

[58] Boogers MM, Chen J, Bax JJ. Myocardial perfusion single photon emission computed tomography for the assessment of mechanical dyssynchrony. *Curr Opin Cardiol*. 2008 Sep;23(5):431-9.

[59] Trimble MA, Borges-Neto S, Velazquez EJ, Chen J, Shaw LK, Pagnanelli R, Garcia EV, Iskandrian AE. Emerging role of myocardial perfusion imaging to evaluate

patients for cardiac resynchronization therapy. *Am J Cardiol.* 2008 Jul 15;102(2):211-7.

[60] Nguyen PL, Trofimov A, Zietman AL. Proton-beam vs intensity-modulated radiation therapy. Which is best for treating prostate cancer? *Oncology (Williston Park).* 2008 Jun;22(7):748-54.

[61] Suit H, Kooy H, Trofimov A, Farr J, Munzenrider J, DeLaney T, Loeffler J, Clasie B, Safai S, Paganetti H. Should positive phase III clinical trial data be required before proton beam therapy is more widely adopted? *No. Radiother Oncol.* 2008 Feb;86(2):148-53

[62] Schneider U, Lomax A, Pemler P, Besserer J, Ross D, Lombriser N, Kaser-Hotz B. The impact of IMRT and proton radiotherapy on secondary cancer incidence. *Strahlenther Onkol.* 2006 Nov;182(11):647-52.

[63] Konski A, Speier W, Hanlon A, Beck JR, Pollack A. Is proton beam therapy cost effective in the treatment of adenocarcinoma of the prostate? *J Clin Oncol.* 2007 Aug 20;25(24):3603-8.

[64] Mock U, Bogner J, Georg D, Auberger T, Pötter R. Comparative treatment planning on localized prostate carcinoma conformal photon- versus proton-based radiotherapy. *Strahlenther Onkol.* 2005 Jul;181(7):448-55.

[65] Weber DC, Trofimov AV, Delaney TF, Bortfeld T. A treatment planning comparison of intensity modulated photon and proton therapy for paraspinal sarcomas. *Int J Radiat Oncol Biol Phys.* 2004 Apr 1;58(5):1596-606.

[66] DeLaney TF. Clinical proton radiation therapy research at the Francis H. Burr Proton Therapy Center. *Technol Cancer Res Treat.* 2007 Aug;6(4 Suppl):61-6.

[67] Fontenot J, Taddei P, Zheng Y, Mirkovic D, Jordan T, Newhauser W. Equivalent dose and effective dose from stray radiation during passively scattered proton radiotherapy for prostate cancer. *Phys Med Biol.* 2008 Mar 21;53(6):1677-88.

[68] Cella L, Lomax A, Miralbell R. Potential role of intensity modulated proton beams in prostate cancer radiotherapy. *Int J Radiat Oncol Biol Phys.* 2001 Jan 1;49(1):217-23.

[69] Weber DC, Ares C, Lomax AJ, Kurtz JM. Radiation therapy planning with photons and protons for early and advanced breast cancer: an overview. *Radiat Oncol.* 2006 Jul 20;1:22.

[70] Goitein M, Jermann M. The relative costs of proton and X-ray radiation therapy. *Clin Oncol (R Coll Radiol).* 2003 Feb;15(1):S37-50.

[71] Paganetti H, Niemierko A, Ancukiewicz M, Gerweck LE, Goitein M, Loeffler JS, Suit HD. Relative biological effectiveness (RBE) values for proton beam therapy. *Int J Radiat Oncol Biol Phys.* 2002 Jun 1;53(2):407-21.

[72] Weber DC, Bogner J, Verwey J, Georg D, Dieckmann K, Escudé L, Caro M, Pötter R, Goitein G, Lomax AJ, Miralbell R. Proton beam radiotherapy versus fractionated stereotactic radiotherapy for uveal melanomas: A comparative study. *Int J Radiat Oncol Biol Phys.* 2005 Oct 1;63(2):373-84.

Chapter IV

TISSUE ENGINEERING AND MEDICAL BIOPOLYMER APPLICATION

APPLICATION OF ENGINEERING IN BIOLOGY

Engineering is a specific science that focuses mainly on the physical aspect. There are man fields of engineering at present. For example, electrical engineering is a specific branch of engineering dealing with electricity. However, due to the concept of convergence of science, engineering becomes emerged with biological science. Application of engineering in biological science helps jump across the inter-science barrier and brings new advent to the world population. For example, merging between computational engineering and genetics biology brings new science called genomics [1-3], which is the modern blooming science at present. Nanoengineering plus medicine forms nanomedicine which is another present new hope of the world for global health development.

Application of engineering on biology helps explain and manipulate difficult biological question. This can be applied in medicine, which is a branch of biological science. Special forms of medical applications can be seen. One of the most famous application is medical engineering. This involves medical instrumentation as well as other applied engineering for medicine. As mentioned, the usefulness of application of engineering in medicine is very much. It helps from diagnosis, treatment and prevention. In this book, the author focuses content on treatment, therefore, treatment will be focused and applied engineering for treatment in medicine will be mentioned. An important therapeutic application is tissue engineering and medical biopolymer science. The application is useful for reconstructive medicine. Specifically, medical biopolymers are presently used in dentistry and orthopedics. With these applications, it can help manage previously untreatable diseases and conditions. Further details will be further discussed.

CONCEPT OF RECONSTRUCTION AND REGENERATIVE MEDICINE

Reconstruction [4-16] and regenerative medicine [17-24] are specific medical sciences for repairing. Theoretically, a thing needs repairing if it is out of used or impaired. This concept is basic fundamental rule in engineering and can be applied in medicine. Destruction to human beings, at any parts, can be expected and seen in daily life. In nature, catabolism is a kind of metabolism focusing on destruction biomolecules in vivo or destruction. Impairment is the thing that anyone cannot avoid. However, the problem will be existence if there is an excessive destruction. Anatomical disturbance is mainly problematic. This can be due to several insults (physical, chemical and biological types). as a concept, such anatomical destruction might result from rooted underlying, which might start at molecular level as in some inherited gene mutated related disorder or directly occurs at gross level such as accidental injury.

When there is an anatomical defect, loss of function cannot be avoided. It is hard to retain normal physiology if there is an anatomical defect. In medicine, treatment for anatomical defect is required. The first aid to limit destruction is necessary. This form can be easily explained in case of first aid for accidental injury. The first aid aims mainly t save life. The second aim is limitation of destruction. in acute phase, limitation of destruction is necessary because it can be a tertiary prevention, limitation of possible disability consequences. After succeed in acute destruction control, further medical management should be planned.

In the past, severe anatomical usually brought disability. The main practice to cope with this problem is rehabilitation. Rehabilitation is an old medical sceicne. This focuses on recovery of lost function by several means. Physical therapy by physiatist is generally practiced in hospital settings. However, this is the specific tertiary prevention using limiting the loss of organ function due to disability. It does not focus on direct repairing for lost anatomical parts.

To repair lost anatomical part is of interest. With concept of medical regeneration in some lizards, the similar phenomenon is the hope of many physicians coping with this problem. The new medical science, regenerative medicine, is developed. This focuses on regeneration after anatomical loss. There are many reports focusing on regenerative medicine especially for the neurological impairment. The details will be further discussed in the next topic in this chapter. Accompanied with regenerative medicine, reconstructive medicine is also developed. Reconstructive medicine focuses on rearrangment of structure to reuse instead of the lost parts. There are many kinds of present reconstructive surgeries. For example, facial reconstructive surgery is used for some specific facial anomaly especially for frontoethmoidal encephalomeningocele. However, in some cases, reconstructive surgery is used for non therapeutic purpose. The good example is the penile reconstruction or vaginal reconstuction surgeries for lesbians and gays.

Table 1. Some important reports on reconstructive medicine

Authors	Details
Galich et al. [25]	Galich et al. analyzed on the results of reconstructive surgery in 19 patients, suffering vascular malformation of the head region [25].
Ozkan and Ozkan [26]	Ozkan and Ozkan reported on the prefabricated pedicled anterolateral thigh flap for reconstruction of a full-thickness defect of the urethra [26].
Vendemia et al. [27]	Vendemia el reported on nipple areola reconstruction by new surgical technique [27].
Avraham et al. [28]	Avraham et al. reported on microsurgical breast reconstruction [28].
Kanchwala and Bucky [29]	Kanchwala and Bucky reported on optimizing pedicled transverse rectus abdominis muscle flap breast reconstruction [29].
Mesbahi et al. [30]	Mesbahi et al. reported on breast reconstruction with prosthetic implants [30].
Ueda et al. [31]	Ueda et al. reported on functional reconstruction of the upper and lower lips and commissure with a forearm flap combined with a free gracilis muscle transfer [31].
Smit et al. [32]	Smit et al. reported on post operative monitoring of microvascular breast reconstructions using the implantable Cook-Swartz doppler system [32].
Nishida and Shimamura [33]	Nishida and Shimamura studied on methods of reconstruction for bone defect after tumor excision [33]. Nishida and Shimamura concluded that although each technique had its proper advantages and disadvantages, the clinical results were similar to the allograft, and numerous techniques were available as reasonable alternatives for allografts [33].
Seyhan [34]	Seyhan reported on reverse thenar perforator flap for volar hand reconstruction [34].
Salgarello et al. [35]	Salgarello et al. reported on the use of a silicone nipple shield as protective device in nipple reconstruction.
Lin et al. [36]	Lin et al. reported on a new three-dimensional imaging device in facial aesthetic and reconstructive surgery [36].
Stuehmer et al. [37]	Stuehmer et al. reported on intraoperative navigation assisted reconstruction of a maxillo-facial gunshot wound [37]. Stuehmer et al. said that the favorable outcome brought surgeons to recommend the technique of merging comparable CT data for reconstructive planning of bilateral mid-facial fractures [37].
Valentini et al. [38]	Valentini et al. reported diabetes as main risk factor in head and neck reconstructive surgery with free flaps [38].
Egeland et al. [39]	Egeland et al. described the basic principals of facial burn care in the pediatric burn population, with a specific focus on lower-eyelid burn ectropion and oral commissure burn scar contracture leading to microstomia [39].
Oruç et al. [40]	Oruç et al. reported on pulley reconstruction with different materials [40].
Eo et al. [41]	Eo et al. reported on the versatility of the dorsalis pedis compound free flap in hand reconstruction [41].
Kryger et al. [42]	Kryger et al. reported on decreased postoperative pain, narcotic, and antiemetic use after breast reduction using a local anesthetic pain pump [42].
Ibrahim and Salem [43]	Ibrahim and Salem reported on the use of a staged Nagata technique for ear reconstruction in burned ears [43].
Villaret et al. [44]	Villaret et al. reported on quality of life in patients treated for cancer of the oral cavity requiring reconstruction [44]. Villaret et al. found that reconstructive techniques played a crucial role in maintenance of satisfactory quality of life [44].
Isik et al. [45]	Isik et al. reported on nasal reconstruction in a patient with prolidase deficiency syndrome [45].
Gevorgyan and Enepekides [46]	Gevorgyan and Enepekides reported on the utility of microvascular anastomotic devices in head and neck reconstruction [46].
Rad et al. [47]	Rad et al. reported on free DIEP and SIEA breast reconstruction to internal mammary intercostal perforating vessels with arterial microanastomosis using a mechanical coupling device [47].
Nicoletti et al. [48]	Nicoletti et al. reported on a case of bioengineered skin for aesthetic reconstruction of the tip of the nose [48].
Livaoğlu et al. [49]	Livaoğlu et al. reported on reconstruction of full-thickness nasal defect by free anterolateral thigh flap [49].

Some Important Reports on Reconstructive and Regenerative Medicine

A. Some Important Reports on Reconstructive Medicine

There are many reports on reconstructive medicine. Some reported papers will be detailed in Table 1.

B. Some Important Reports on Regenerative Medicine

There are also many reports on regenerative medicine. Some reported reports will be detailed in Table 2.

It can be seen that there are variety of attempt to use of regenerative treatment.

The common focus is on dentistry, cardiology and neurology. The main tool is stem cell. More details on stem cell can be read in another chapter in this book.

Why Anatomical Lost Needs Therapy?

"Why anatomical lost needs therapy"? is the main question to understand before study on tissue engineering. The answer to this question can be

a) Lost of parts means lost or not complete. Function of any parts of human body will be full if it is complete. It is assumed in general that anatomical lost is not equal to functional lost. Functional lost of some organs such as liver and kidney might not be problematic if such lost is not extensive. However, overt anatomical lost is usually problematic and causes functional lost.
b) Lost of parts might bring to more lost. Learning from the case of a building, if there is a defect in its basement or pillar, the collapse of overall building can be expected. This is the same. Loss of some parts of human beings, especially for weight bearing parts can bring the excessive weight stress as a physical insult to other parts and will bring further destruction and finally results in lost.
c) Treatment of lost is fit to the concept of clinical rehabilitation practice. Treatment can be helpful as tertiary prevention for extensive disability.
d) In some cases, lost means ugly appearance. This is a big psychological effect to mind. In cosmetic medicine, treatment for anatomical lost is the core. The important affected parts to be concerned are the face, tooth and limbs.

In the past, treatment for anatomical lost might be done but not specific. Application of prosthesis can be used but it is not as good as real parts. There are several attempts to find a better alternative and this leads to the emerging of tissue engineering.

Table 2. Some important reports on regenerative medicine

Authors	Details
Nishikii et al. [50]	Nishikii et al. found that etalloproteinase regulation improves in vitro generation of efficacious platelets from mouse embryonic stem cells [50].
Datal and Lee [51]	Datal and Lee reported on treatment of burn injury by cellular repair [51].
Yamahara and Nagaya [52]	Yamahara and Nagaya reported on stem cell implantation for myocardial disorders [52].
Jubel et al. [53]	Jubel et al. reported on transplantation of de novo scaffold-free cartilage implants into sheep knee chondral defects [53].
Nieponice et al. [54]	Nieponice et al. reported on an extracellular matrix scaffold for esophageal stricture prevention after circumferential EMR [54].
Toyoda et al. [55]	Toyoda et al. reported on myogenic transdifferentiation of menstrual blood-derived cells [55].
Jentsch and Purschwitz [56]	Jentsch and Purschwitz performed a clinical study evaluating the treatment of supra-alveolar-type defects with access flap surgery with and without an enamel matrix protein derivative [56].
Rovó and Gratwohl [57]	Rovó and Gratwohl reported on plasticity after allogeneic hematopoietic stem cell transplantation [57]. Rovó and Gratwohl metanalyzed on the published data on non-hematopoietic chimerism, donor cell contribution to tissue repair, the controversies related to the methods used to detect donor-derived non-hematopoietic cells and the functional impact of this phenomenon in diverse specific target tissues and organs in this work [57].
Trope [58]	Trope studied on regenerative potential of dental pulp [58].
López Moratalla [59]	López Moratalla discussed on ethics for regenerative therapy [59]. López Moratalla said that it was an ethical commitment of the scientific community to give serious and precise information about the advances, problems and solutions involved an regenerative treatment [59].
Romanos and Nentwig [60]	Romanos and Nentwig reported on regenerative therapy of deep peri-implant infrabony defects after CO2 laser implant surface decontamination [60].
Connonly [61]	Connonly et al. reported on cavernous nerve regeneration using acellular nerve grafts [61].
Levey et al. [62]	Levy et al. reported on regenerative effect of neural-induced human mesenchymal stromal cells in rat models of Parkinson's disease [62].
van-Larr and Tyndall [63]	van Laar and Tyndall reported on cellular therapy of systemic sclerosis [63]. van Laar and Tyndall proposed that therapies involving mesenchymal stromal cells had to be studied in clinical settings because of their anti-inflammatory and tissue regenerative properties and their favorable risk/benefit ratio [63].
Atouri et al. [64]	Atouri et al. reported on myocardial regenerative treatment [64]. Atouri et al. reported that use of autologous donor cells was more preferred to avoid immune rejection [64].
van Vliet et al. [65]	van Vliet et al. reported that progenitor cells isolated from the human heart was a potential cell source for regenerative therapy [65]. van Vliet et al. said that human cardiomyocyte pogenitors which were localiszd within the atria, atrioventricular region, and epicardial layer of the octal and adult human heart were the good tool for regenerative therapy [65].

TISSUE ENGINEERING

Tissue engineering is a medical science manipulating with tissue [66-68]. The main areas of tissue engineering are for treatment of anatomical lost. The tissue engineering makes used of cell regeneration plus biomaterial application. The concept can be easily explained as the application of cement on the wire for building up a building. This is probable but there are still some problems to be mentioned as will be further detailed. The conditions to be fulfilled are

a) The repair is for the anatomical lost that has functional problem (as previously mentioned).
b) There is a need to repair.
c) Preparation of the site is necessary.
d) In repairing there should be core structure. This usually makes use of special biomolecules. Similar to construction of a building, there must be a core as steal for cement attachment.

There are brief steps that seem easy but very difficult in real practice. There are many problems of tissue engineering. How to succeed in taking care of the graft to survive is the big problem. It should be noted that cell is a living thing, not cement, needs proper condition to maintain viability. Usually cell death after engraftment is due to poor oxygenation, which might relate to poor designing of biomaterial cores. The proper ratio needs further researches to explain. Bonfield said that the particular requirements of tissue-engineering scaffolds with respect to macro- and micro-porosity, as well as chemistry must be focused in designing [68]. Bonfield noted that the subsequent integration and longevity of the implanted device was based on the effectiveness of the associated biological repair [68]. However, using a concept of nanomedicine, good biomedical core must have intermolecular space that allows cell attachment and perfusion of necessary substances for cellular metabolisms especially oxygen for cell viability.

There are also many reports on tissue engineering. Some reported reports will be detailed in Table 3.

Medical Biopolymer Application

Application of polymer science in medicine is acceptable for its usefulness. With advent on polymer science, there are many new adapted polymers for medical usage. Indeed, this field was well developed in dentistry. There are many biomaterials in presently used. However, the next generation is the application for tissue engineering and regenerative medicine. Important examples will be hereby presented.

- Atelocollagen

  Atelocollagen is accepted as a potential carrier of therapeutics [79]. Basically, collagen is abundant and makes up about 25% of the total protein in animal organisms [79]. Atelecollagen is a major product of the digestion of collagen type I, which was used for the first time in tissue engineering already in the 1970s [79]. Atelocollagen is accepted in medical science an optimal vehicle to transport medication which may be used in vivo with very limited risk [79].

- Elastin

  Elastic is another important structural protein. Daamen et al. noted that elastin could be applied in biomaterials in several forms, including insoluble elastin fibres, hydrolysed soluble elastin, recombinant tropoelastin, repeats of synthetic peptide sequences and as block copolymers of elastin, possibly in combination with other biopolymers [80].

- Hyaluronic acid

Hyaluronic acid is a natural biopolymer with a broad range of biomedical and industrial applications [81]. In clinical medicine, it can be used in certain ophthalmological and otological surgeries and cosmetic regeneration and reconstruction of soft tissue [81].

Table 3. Some important reports on tissue engineering

Authors	Details
Yamzon et al. [69]	Yamzon et al. reported on current status of tissue engineering in pediatric urology [69]. Yamzon et al. said that clinical trials might lead to transforming reconstructive surgery as well as current surgical practice in patients with neurogenic bladders and urinary incontinence [69].
Yamamiya et al. [70]	Yamamiya et al. reported on tissue-engineered cultured periosteum used with platelet-rich plasma and hydroxyapatite in treating human osseous defects [70]. Yamamiya et al. reported that treatment with a combination of human cultured periosteum sheets, platelet-rich plasma, and porous hydroxyapatite led to a significantly more favorable clinical improvement in infrabony periodontal defects [70].
Vavken et al. [71]	Vavken et al. reported on tissue engineering in orthopaedic surgery [71]. Vavken et al. found that autologous chondrocyte transplantation was an expensive and complex procedure [71]. In addition, in direct comparison with alternative treatments autologous chondrocyte transplantation produces could yield at least as good in the short-term, and most likely better in the long-term due to the high quality repairing [71].
Jawad et al. [72]	Jawad et al. reviewed on myocardial tissue engineering [72]. Jawad et al. proposed that many different cell types including include both autologous and embryonic stem cells could be used for cell therapy and myocardial tissue engineering [72].
Mohammadi et al. [73]	Mohammadi et al. reported on culture of human gingival fibroblasts on a biodegradable scaffold and evaluation of its effect on attached gingival [73]. Mohammadi et al. concluded that the tissue-engineered mucosal graft was safe and capable of generating keratinized tissue [73].
Liu et al. [74]	Liu et al. reported on optimal combination of soluble factors for tissue engineering of permanent cartilage from cultured human chondrocytes [74]. Liu et al. concluded that bone morphogenetic protein-2 and insulin plus triiodothyronine was the optimal combination to regenerate a clinically practical permanent cartilage from autologous chondrocytes [74].
Hollander et al. [75]	Hollander et al. reported on maturation of tissue engineered cartilage implanted in injured and osteoarthritic human knees [75]. Hollander et al. concluded that cartilage injuries could be effectively repaired using tissue engineering, and osteoarthritis could not inhibit the regeneration process [75].
Ferrari et al. [76]	Ferrari et al. reviewed on gene therapy in combination with tissue engineering to treat epidermolysis bullosa [76].
Giraud et al. [77]	Giraud et al. engineered a biodegradable skeletal muscle graft (ESMG) tissue and investigated its functional effect after implantation on the epicardium of an infarcted heart segment [77]. Giraud et al. found that it was probable to improve systolic heart function following myocardial infarction through implantation of differentiated muscle fibers seeded on a gel-type scaffold despite a low rate of survival [77].
Ndreu et al. [78]	Ndreu et al. reported on electrospun biodegradable nanofibrous mats for tissue engineering [78]. Ndruc et al. concluded that scaffolds prepared by electrospinning had high potential for use in further studies leading to bone tissue engineering applications [78].

REFERENCES

[1] Mychaleckyj JC. Genome mapping statistics and bioinformatics. *Methods Mol Biol.* 2007;404:461-88.

[2] Liao G, Zhang X, Clark DJ, Peltz G. A genomic "roadmap" to "better" drugs. *Drug Metab Rev.* 2008;40(2):225-39.

[3] Tanaka H. Bioinformatics and genomics for opening new perspective for personalized care. *Stud Health Technol Inform.* 2008;134:47-58.

[4] Blackburn VF, Blackburn AV. Taking a history in aesthetic surgery: SAGA--the surgeon's tool for patient selection. *J Plast Reconstr Aesthet Surg.* 2008 Jul;61(7):723-9.

[5] Loiselle F, Mahabir RC, Harrop AR. Levels of evidence in plastic surgery research over 20 years. *Plast Reconstr Surg.* 2008 Apr;121(4):207e-11e.

[6] Engell-Nørregård L, Sørensen J. The bilobed flap: reconstruction of nasal and extra-nasal skin defect. *Ugeskr Laeger.* 2007 Dec 10;169(50):4337-40.

[7] Moore AM. The section on plastic and reconstructive surgery in review. *South Med J.* 1967 Mar;60(3):327-8.

[8] Antognini F, Cavina C, Giuliani R, Caradonna V. Anesthesiological problems in maxillo-facial surgical interventions and reconstructive plastic surgery] *Minerva Stomatol.* 1977 Oct-Dec;26(4):155-73.

[9] Glicenstein J. From the French Society of Plastic and Reconstructive Surgery to the French Society of Plastic Reconstructive and Aesthetic Surgery. *Ann Chir Plast Esthet.* 2004 Apr;49(2):81-88

[10] Aufricht G. Story of the foundation of the Plastic and Reconstructive Surgery journal and reminiscences of the early formative years of plastic surgery as a specialty. *Plast Reconstr Surg.* 1981 Sep;68(3):370-5.

[11] Fredricks S. History of the American Society of Plastic and Reconstructive Surgeons. *Plast Reconstr Surg.* 1995 May;95(6):1135.

[12] Pizzo AJ. The history of the Southeastern Society of Plastic and Reconstructive Surgeons. *Ann Plast Surg.* 1999 Jan;42(1):1-6

[13] Schnur PL. History of the American Society of Plastic and Reconstructive Surgeons, Inc., 1931-1994: technical corrections. *Plast Reconstr Surg.* 1995 Jun;95(7):1332-3.

[14] Paletta FX. History of the American Society of Plastic and Reconstructive Surgeons, Inc., 1931-1981: its growth, change, unity. *Plast Reconstr Surg.* 1981 Sep;68(3):292-369.

[15] Lynch JB. Five-year history of the American Society of Plastic and Reconstructive Surgeons, 1974--1978. *Plast Reconstr Surg.* 1979 Jun;63(6):800-11.

[16] Marino H. Reminiscences of the American Society of Plastic and Reconstructive Surgeons, Inc., and some of its members. *Plast Reconstr Surg.* 1981 Sep;68(3):376-80.

[17] Sakurada K, McDonald FM, Shimada F. Regenerative medicine and stem cell based drug discovery. *Angew Chem Int Ed Engl.* 2008;47(31):5718-38.

[18] Winkler DA. Network models in drug discovery and regenerative medicine. *Biotechnol Annu Rev.* 2008;14:143-70.

[19] Nolan K, Millet Y, Ricordi C, Stabler CL. Tissue engineering and biomaterials in regenerative medicine. *Cell Transplant.* 2008;17(3):241-3.

[20] Bajada S, Mazakova I, Richardson JB, Ashammakhi N. Updates on stem cells and their applications in regenerative medicine. *J Tissue Eng Regen Med.* 2008 Jun;2(4):169-83.

[21] Gurtner GC, Werner S, Barrandon Y, Longaker MT. Wound repair and regeneration. *Nature.* 2008 May 15;453(7193):314-21.

[22] Xu Y, Shi Y, Ding S. A chemical approach to stem-cell biology and regenerative medicine. *Nature.* 2008 May 15;453(7193):338-44.

[23] Miyake J. Social effects in regenerative medicine. *Nippon Rinsho.* 2008 May;66(5):1004-12.

[24] Ida R. Ethical, legal and social issues in regenerative medicine. *Nippon Rinsho.* 2008 May;66(5):991-7.

[25] Galich SP, Chernukha LM, Dabizha AY, Furmanov AY, Reznikov AV, Ahltman IV. Possibilities of reconstructive plastic surgery in the treatment of vascular malformations of the head region. *Klin Khir.* 2008 Mar;(3):23-7.

[26] Ozkan O, Ozkan O. The prefabricated pedicled anterolateral thigh flap for reconstruction of a full-thickness defect of the urethra. *J Plast Reconstr Aesthet Surg.* 2008 Aug 2. [Epub ahead of print]

[27] Vendemia N, Mesbahi AN, McCarthy CM, Disa JJ. Nipple areola reconstruction. *Cancer J.* 2008 Jul-Aug;14(4):253-7.

[28] Avraham T, Clavin N, Mehrara BJ. Microsurgical breast reconstruction. *Cancer J.* 2008 Jul-Aug;14(4):241-7.

[29] Kanchwala SK, Bucky LP. Optimizing pedicled transverse rectus abdominis muscle flap breast reconstruction. *Cancer J.* 2008 Jul-Aug;14(4):236-40.

[30] Mesbahi AN, McCarthy CM, Disa JJ. Breast reconstruction with prosthetic implants. *Cancer J.* 2008 Jul-Aug;14(4):230-5.

[31] Ueda K, Oba S, Nakai K, Okada M, Kurokawa N, Nuri T. Functional reconstruction of the upper and lower lips and commissure with a forearm flap combined with a free gracilis muscle transfer. *J Plast Reconstr Aesthet Surg.* 2008 Jul 25. [Epub ahead of print]

[32] Smit JM, Whitaker IS, Liss AG, Audolfsson T, Kildal M, Acosta R. Post operative monitoring of microvascular breast reconstructions using the implantable Cook-Swartz doppler system: A study of 145 probes & technical discussion. *J Plast Reconstr Aesthet Surg.* 2008 Jul 31. [Epub ahead of print]

[33] Nishida J, Shimamura T. Methods of reconstruction for bone defect after tumor excision: A review of alternatives. *Med Sci Monit.* 2008 Aug;14(8):RA107-113.

[34] Seyhan T. Reverse thenar perforator flap for volar hand reconstruction. *J Plast Reconstr Aesthet Surg.* 2008 Jul 28. [Epub ahead of print]

[35] Salgarello M, Cervelli D, Barone-Adesi L. The use of a silicone nipple shield as protective device in nipple reconstruction. *J Plast Reconstr Aesthet Surg.* 2008 Jul 23. [Epub ahead of print]

[36] Lin SJ, Patel N, O'Shaughnessy K, Fine N. A new three-dimensional imaging device in facial aesthetic and reconstructive surgery. *Otolaryngol Head Neck Surg*. 2008 Aug;139(2):313-5.

[37] Stuehmer C, Essig H, Schramm A, Rücker M, Eckardt A, Gellrich NC. Intraoperative navigation assisted reconstruction of a maxillo-facial gunshot wound. *Oral Maxillofac Surg*. 2008 Jul 25. [Epub ahead of print]

[38] Valentini V, Cassoni A, Marianetti TM, Mitro V, Gennaro P, Ialongo C, Iannetti G. Diabetes as main risk factor in head and neck reconstructive surgery with free flaps. *J Craniofac Surg*. 2008 Jul;19(4):1080-4.

[39] Egeland B, More S, Buchman SR, Cederna PS. Management of difficult pediatric facial burns: reconstruction of burn-related lower eyelid ectropion and perioral contractures. *J Craniofac Surg*. 2008 Jul;19(4):960-9.

[40] Oruç M, Ulusoy MG, Kankaya Y, Koçer U, Serbetçi K, Hasrc N. Pulley reconstruction with different materials: experimental study. *Ann Plast Surg*. 2008 Aug;61(2):215-20.

[41] Eo S, Kim Y, Kim JY, Oh S. The versatility of the dorsalis pedis compound free flap in hand reconstruction. *Ann Plast Surg*. 2008 Aug;61(2):157-63.

[42] Kryger ZB, Rawlani V, Lu L, Fine NA. Decreased postoperative pain, narcotic, and antiemetic use after breast reduction using a local anesthetic pain pump. *Ann Plast Surg*. 2008 Aug;61(2):147-52.

[43] Ibrahim SM, Salem IL. Burned ear: the use of a staged Nagata technique for ear reconstruction. *J Plast Reconstr Aesthet Surg*. 2008 Jul 21.

[44] Villaret AB, Cappiello J, Piazza C, Pedruzzi B, Nicolai P. Quality of life in patients treated for cancer of the oral cavity requiring reconstruction: a prospective study. *Acta Otorhinolaryngol Ital*. 2008 Jun;28(3):120-5.

[45] Isik D, Bekerecioglu M, Mutaf M. Nasal reconstruction in a patient with prolidase deficiency syndrome. *J Plast Reconstr Aesthet Surg*. 2008 Jul 16. [Epub ahead of print]

[46] Gevorgyan A, Enepekides DJ. The utility of microvascular anastomotic devices in head and neck reconstruction. *Curr Opin Otolaryngol Head Neck Surg*. 2008 Aug;16(4):331-4.

[47] Rad AN, Flores JI, Rosson GD. Free DIEP and SIEA breast reconstruction to internal mammary intercostal perforating vessels with arterial microanastomosis using a mechanical coupling device. *Microsurgery*. 2008 Jul 11. [Epub ahead of print]

[48] Nicoletti G, Scevola S, Faga A. Bioengineered Skin for Aesthetic Reconstruction of the Tip of the Nose: A Case Report. *Dermatol Surg*. 2008 Jun 27. [Epub ahead of print]

[49] Livaoğlu M, Karacal N, Bektas D, Bahadir O. Reconstruction of full-thickness nasal defect by free anterolateral thigh flap. *Acta Otolaryngol*. 2008 Jul 7:1-4. [Epub ahead of print]

[50] Nishikii H, Eto K, Tamura N, Hattori K, Heissig B, Kanaji T, Sawaguchi A, Goto S, Ware J, Nakauchi H. Metalloproteinase regulation improves in vitro generation of efficacious platelets from mouse embryonic stem cells. *J Exp Med*. 2008 Aug 4;205(8):1917-27.

[51] Dalal ND, Lee RC. Treatment of burn injury by cellular repair. *J Craniofac Surg.* 2008 Jul;19(4):903-6.

[52] Yamahara K, Nagaya N. Stem cell implantation for myocardial disorders. *Curr Drug Deliv.* 2008 Jul;5(3):224-9.

[53] Jubel A, Andermahr J, Schiffer G, Fischer J, Rehm KE, Stoddart MJ, Häuselmann HJ. Transplantation of de novo scaffold-free cartilage implants into sheep knee chondral defects. *Am J Sports Med.* 2008 Aug;36(8):1555-64.

[54] Nieponice A, McGrath K, Qureshi I, Beckman EJ, Luketich JD, Gilbert TW, Badylak SF. An extracellular matrix scaffold for esophageal stricture prevention after circumferential EMR. *Gastrointest Endosc.* 2008 Jul 25. [Epub ahead of print]

[55] Toyoda M, Cui Ch, Umezawa A. Myogenic transdifferentiation of menstrual blood-derived cells. *Acta Myol.* 2007 Dec;26(3):176-8.

[56] Jentsch H, Purschwitz R. A clinical study evaluating the treatment of supra-alveolar-type defects with access flap surgery with and without an enamel matrix protein derivative: a pilot study. *J Clin Periodontol.* 2008 Jun 24. [Epub ahead of print]

[57] Rovó A, Gratwohl A. Plasticity after allogeneic hematopoietic stem cell transplantation. *Biol Chem.* 2008 Jul;389(7):825-36.

[58] Trope M. Regenerative potential of dental pulp. *Pediatr Dent.* 2008 May-Jun;30(3):206-10.

[59] López Moratalla N. Ethical Principles in Research related to Regenerative Therapy. *Cuad Bioet.* 2008 May-Aug;19(66):195-210.

[60] Romanos GE, Nentwig GH. Regenerative therapy of deep peri-implant infrabony defects after CO2 laser implant surface decontamination. *Int J Periodontics Restorative Dent.* 2008 Jun;28(3):245-55.

[61] Connolly SS, Yoo JJ, Abouheba M, Soker S, McDougal WS, Atala A. Cavernous nerve regeneration using acellular nerve grafts. *World J Urol.* 2008 Jul 2. [Epub ahead of print]

[62] Levy YS, Bahat-Stroomza M, Barzilay R, Burshtein A, Bulvik S, Barhum Y, Panet H, Melamed E, Offen D. Regenerative effect of neural-induced human mesenchymal stromal cells in rat models of Parkinson's disease. *Cytotherapy.* 2008;10(4):340-52.

[63] van Laar JM, Tyndall A. Cellular therapy of systemic sclerosis. *Curr Rheumatol Rep.* 2008 Jul;10(3):189-94.

[64] Atoui R, Shum-Tim D, Chiu RC. Myocardial regenerative therapy: immunologic basis for the potential "universal donor cells". *Ann Thorac Surg.* 2008 Jul;86(1):327-34.

[65] van Vliet P, Roccio M, Smits AM, van Oorschot AA, Metz CH, van Veen TA, Sluijter JP, Doevendans PA, Goumans MJ. Progenitor cells isolated from the human heart: a potential cell source for regenerative therapy. *Neth Heart J.* 2008 May;16(5):163-9.

[66] Nolan K, Millet Y, Ricordi C, Stabler CL. Tissue engineering and biomaterials in regenerative medicine. *Cell Transplant.* 2008;17(3):241-3.

[67] Spector M. Biomaterials-based tissue engineering and regenerative medicine solutions to musculoskeletal problems. *Swiss Med Wkly.* 2006 May 13;136(19-20):293-301.

[68] Bonfield W. Designing porous scaffolds for tissue engineering. *Philos Transact A Math Phys Eng Sci.* 2006 Jan 15;364(1838):227-32.

[69] Yamzon J, Perin L, Koh CJ. Current status of tissue engineering in pediatric urology. *Curr Opin Urol.* 2008 Jul;18(4):404-7.

[70] Yamamiya K, Okuda K, Kawase T, Hata K, Wolff LF, Yoshie H. Tissue-engineered cultured periosteum used with platelet-rich plasma and hydroxyapatite in treating human osseous defects. *J Periodontol.* 2008 May;79(5):811-8.

[71] Vavken P, Gruber M, Dorotka R. Tissue engineering in orthopaedic surgery--clinical effectiveness and cost effectiveness of autologous chondrocyte transplantation. *Z Orthop Unfall.* 2008 Jan-Feb;146(1):26-30

[72] Jawad H, Ali NN, Lyon AR, Chen QZ, Harding SE, Boccaccini AR. Myocardial tissue engineering: a review. *J Tissue Eng Regen Med.* 2007 Sep-Oct;1(5):327-42.

[73] Mohammadi M, Shokrgozar MA, Mofid R. Culture of human gingival fibroblasts on a biodegradable scaffold and evaluation of its effect on attached gingiva: a randomized, controlled pilot study. *J Periodontol.* 2007 Oct;78(10):1897-903.

[74] Liu G, Kawaguchi H, Ogasawara T, Asawa Y, Kishimoto J, Takahashi T, Chung UI, Yamaoka H, Asato H, Nakamura K, Takato T, Hoshi K. Optimal combination of soluble factors for tissue engineering of permanent cartilage from cultured human chondrocytes. *J Biol Chem.* 2007 Jul 13;282(28):20407-15.

[75] Hollander AP, Dickinson SC, Sims TJ, Brun P, Cortivo R, Kon E, Marcacci M, Zanasi S, Borrione A, De Luca C, Pavesio A, Soranzo C, Abatangelo G. Maturation of tissue engineered cartilage implanted in injured and osteoarthritic human knees. *Tissue Eng.* 2006 Jul;12(7):1787-98.

[76] Ferrari S, Pellegrini G, Matsui T, Mavilio F, De Luca M. Gene therapy in combination with tissue engineering to treat epidermolysis bullosa. *Expert Opin Biol Ther.* 2006 Apr;6(4):367-78.

[77] Giraud MN, Ayuni E, Cook S, Siepe M, Carrel TP, Tevaearai HT. Hydrogel-based Engineered Skeletal Muscle Grafts Normalize Heart Function Early After Myocardial Infarction. *Artif Organs.* 2008 Jul 30. [Epub ahead of print]

[78] Ndreu A, Nikkola L, Ylikauppila H, Ashammakhi N, Hasirci V. Electrospun biodegradable nanofibrous mats for tissue engineering. *Nanomed.* 2008 Feb;3(1):45-60.

[79] Wysocki T, Sacewicz I, Wiktorska M, Niewiarowska J. Atelocollagen as a potential carrier of therapeutics. *Postepy Hig Med Dosw (Online).* 2007 Nov 5;61:646-54.

[80] Daamen WF, Veerkamp JH, van Hest JC, van Kuppevelt TH. Elastin as a biomaterial for tissue engineering. *Biomaterials.* 2007 Oct;28(30):4378-98.

[81] Kogan G, Soltés L, Stern R, Gemeiner P. Hyaluronic acid: a natural biopolymer with a broad range of biomedical and industrial applications. *Biotechnol Lett.* 2007 Jan;29(1):17-25.

Chapter V

TRANSPLANTATION IN MEDICINE

TRANSPLANTATION: WHAT IS IT?

When an organ lost, it is necessary to get medical management. Organ lost usually means lost of function. In severe case, organ lost ends up with death. There is no method to recover in the past and this has been continuously searched for the solution. Transplantation is a new concept using the replacement of the lost organs by the new ones. New ones means new organ from the others. Therefore, it means transferring of one's organ to another. This is ethical concern and new concept in medicine. Indeed, organ transplantation has long history. More than 50 years are recorded [1-3]. Learning of history of transplantation is necessary to allow us to appreciate the great potential offered by current biomedical science and engineering for future developments in the therapies of this more than natural practice [2-3]. At present, embryonic stem cells are used in the studies of the differentiation of various cells or tissues for transplantation therapy, because of their pluripotential property to differentiate into almost all types of cells in the body [1].

BEFORE TRANSPLANTATION

Transplantation should be set as the final choice of treatment. Indeed, transplantation is usually indicated if there is no other choice of treatment. It is usually decided in cases of end stage of disease such as kidney failure. Transplantation is a high cost treatment and complicated. It required a good inclusion of patients. There must be a good system to include or select the patient for transplantation. It is needed to classify whether a case is proper for transplantation or not. This must rely on many factors. Expectation of succeed should be the main factor for making decision. Because transplantation also seems high risk and this usually brings death to the patient earlier than without transplantation condition. After good preparation, a patient will be finalized for appropriateness for transplantation.

Another fact to be concerned is how to find organ for transplantation. Organ donation is the accepted way. However, other ways such as selling and stealing are possible but these methods should be and must be banned. Organ donation center can be seen in many big cities. Many organ centers cannot get sufficient amount of donated organs. How to cope with this problem is needed. In general, the basic organ donation is eye donation for corneal transplantation. The other organs can be sporadically donated. A closed related donation to organ donation is cadaver donation for medical education. This is done in some specific countries such as Thailand but is not permitted in many Islamic countries. This can be another source of organ donation. It should be noted for some fact from donation center. There are some believes that can prevent donation. There are also some conditions that prevent donation. Thos condition were well described the report by Agthong and Wiwanitkit [4]. The HIV seropositive is an important condition prevention donation or usage of donated organ for further transplantation [5]. Screening for infectious disease especially viral borne diseases should be done for all donors [6]. Some important reports on infectious diseases transmitted by organ transplantation will be presented and discussed in Table 1.

To help reader more appreciate on this topic, the author hereby focuses on a very specific situation *Pseudallescheria boydii* brain abscess. systemic scedosporiasis due to the anamorph or asexual form *Pseudallescheria boydii* (*Scedosporium apiospermum*) has become an important cause of opportunistic mycosis, especially in patients undergoing high-risk hematopoietic stem cell transplantation [21]. It can be mistaken, histologically, for *Aspergillus* Spp. However, *P. boydii* is clinically distinguished by resistance to most antifungals and its ability to cause invasive mycoses in immunocompetent patients. There are at least 26 reported cases of *P. boydii* brain abscesses from 1965 to 2007 with only four survivors. The last case is in Thailand: a famous singer got this infection, still in the hospital, and becomes a well-known topic for the general population as well as the most famous infected case [22]. From the literatures, there are two groups of patients, a) the immunocompromised subjects, especially for those who got transplantation and b) the immunocompetent subjects with the history of near drowning. Most cases usually developed CNS symptoms gradually as the nature of CNS fungal infection [23-24]. The recent widely used antifungal, which mentioned for effective therapeutic effect, is voriconazole [23]. Due to the widely practiced transplantation and the dirty contaminated water in the city drainage at the present day, the risk of getting this infection might be higher than the past. The awareness of this infection, which can lead to early diagnosis and prompt treatment, is necessary.

In addition to screening for infectious agent, another basic screening is for matching between donor and recipient. This is also similar to basic cross matching used in classical transfusion medicine. However, the screening for transplantation is more complex. There is a specific set of laboratory investigation for matching test in transplantation medicine. An interesting example of laboratory investigation is human leukocyte antigen (HLA) typing [25]. This is routinely indicated for all cases aiming at organ transplantation procedure. Little said that there were a number of different approaches that could be made in order to achieve HLA type depending on the number of samples being processed, the level of resolution to be achieved, and the cost of providing the various tests [25]. The World Marrow Donor Association recently proposed guidelines for establishing the extent and quality of histocompatibility testing for unrelated donor registries, umbilical cord blood banks, and transplant centers involved in international exchange of hematopoietic stem cells for allogeneic transplantation and this guideline is presently acceptable in transplant medicine [26]. According to this guideline, quality assurance and quality control for HLA testing, and construction for the format of the HLA database of donor types are also necessary for accreditation [26].

Table 1. Some interesting reports on infectious disease transmitted by organ transplantation

Authors	Details
CDC [7]	USA CDC reported on transplantation-transmitted tuberculosis [6]. USA CDC noted that organ recovery personnel should consider risk factors for TB when assessing all organ donors to reduce the risk for tubercuolosis transmission associated with organ transplantation [7].
Hassan et al. [8]	Hassan et al. reported on infectious disease risk factors of corneal graft donors [8]. Hassan et al. said that corneal grafts with eye tissue obtained from donors dying in the hospital or with cancer might have an increased risk of postsurgical endophthalmitis, possibly due to donor-to-host microbial transmission [8]. Hassan noted that improvements in microbiological control could decrease infection associated with corneal transplant [8].
Palacios et al. [9]	Palacios et al. reported on arenavirus transmitted through solid-organ transplantation [9]. They reported on three cases receiving visceral-organ transplants from a single donor on the same day died of a febrile illness 4 to 6 weeks after transplantation [9].
Gajewska et al. [10]	Gajewska et al. reported that the occurrence of HPV infections with pregnant renal transplant recipients in comparison with normal pregnancy was on similar level, however, high percentage of HPV transmission from mother to neonate was obtained [10].
Kumar and Humar [11]	Kumar and Humar reviewed on pandemic influenza and its implications for transplantation [11].
Zöllner et al. [12]	Zöllner et al. reported on clinical reactivation after liver transplantation with an unusual minor strain of hepatitis B virus in an occult carrier [12].
Campos et al. [13]	Campos et al. reported on bacterial and fungal pneumonias after lung transplantation. Campos et al. found that bacterial and fungal infections were frequent and contribute to higher mortality in lung transplant recipients and *Pseudomonas aeruginosa* was the most frequent agent of respiratory infections [13].
Chrastina et al. [14]	Chrastina et al. reported on cytomegalovirus (CMV) infection and CMV disease in kidney transplant recipients [14].
Mattner et al. [15]	Mattner et al. reported on an adenovirus type F41 outbreak in a pediatric bone marrow transplant unit [15]. Mattner et al. reported that adenovirus was identified in blood and stool specimens from 6 children on a pediatric bone marrow transplant unit within 2 weeks in this epidemic [15].
Nordquist and Aronson [16]	Nordquist and Aronson reported on Pyogranulomatous cystitis associated with *Toxoplasma gondii* infection in a cat after renal transplantation [16].
Alkhunaizi et al. [17]	Alkhunaizi et al. reported on transfusion-transmitted malaria in a kidney transplant recipient [17].
Schmoldt et al. [18]	Schmoldt et al. reported on molecular evidence of nosocomial Pneumocystis jirovecii transmission among 16 patients after kidney transplantation [18].
Yilmaz et al. [19]	Yilmaz et al. reported on Burkitt's lymphoma following a pediatric liver transplantation [19].
Waldman and Kopp [20]	Waldman and Kopp reported on Parvovirus-B19-associated complications in renal transplant recipients [20].

There are also other sets of laboratory investigation in transplantation medicine. Because organ transplantation recipient must rely on immunosuppressive drug for life long after transplantation they are accepted as immunocompromised subjects. A test for any possible problematic opportunistic infection is needed. These usually included Chest X ray, tuberculin test, sputum examination, stool examination and CMV antibody test. Important reports on opportunistic infections after organ transplantation are already summarized and presented in Table 1. From Table 1, the readers can see that there are several problems that can be seen after organ transplantation. This verifies the necessity of previously mentioned concept to weight between risk and benefit of transplantation for each case before real transplantation.

ORGAN TRANSPLANTATION

A. Heart Transplantation

Table 2. Some interesting reports on heart transplantation

Authors	Details
Lehmkuhl et al. [37]	Lehmkuhl et al. reported on enteric-coated mycophenolate-sodium usage in heart transplantation [37]. Lehmkuhl et al. concluded that this administration was useful [37].
Quarta et al. [38]	Quarta et al. reported on safety and efficacy of ezetimibe with low doses of simvastatin in heart transplant recipients [38].
Potena et al. [39]	Potena et al. reported on long-term effect of folic acid therapy in heart transplant recipients [39]. Potena et al. concluded that it was proper to apply folate therapy to heart transplant recipients and it was feasible that properties other than homocysteine reduction might provide antitumoral benefits [39].
Singh et al. [40]	Singh et al. reported on treatment of recurrent chest pain in a heart transplant recipient using spinal cord stimulation [40].
Letsas et al. [41]	Letsas et al. reported on catheter ablation of recipient-to-donor atrioatrial conduction with wenckebach-like phenomenon after orthotopic heart transplantation [41].
Lacy et al. [42]	Lacy et al. reported on autologous stem cell transplant after heart transplant for light chain amyloid cardiomyopathy [42].
Marelli et al. [43]	Marelli et al. reported on long-term outcomes of heart transplantation in older recipients [43]. Marelli et al. reported that the increased risk of renal failure and malignancy among elderly patients influenced the survival rate [43].

Heart transplantation is an organ transplantation at the early phase [27]. Beginning with an isolated heart transplant performed as a technical exercise in 1905, slowly accumulated experimental efforts provided answers to several queries involving technique, recipient and graft protection, post-transplant function and immunology, and provided a foundation for subsequent clinical applications [28-29]. Most notable is the Stanford team, organized by Dr. Norman Shumway, who continued to transplant human hearts when other institutions had abandoned hope and because of the commitment of that team, cardiac transplantation has become successful [28-30]. The practice of pediatric heart transplantation was developed later than the adult ones. Similar process has been passed for years [29]. Karpawich said that as pacing techniques were used in younger patients, clinical improvements, comparable to older adult patients, even delaying heart transplant, might be anticipated [31]. Law said that clinical cardiology needed further improvement to assess organ dysfunction and to correlate these methods to early graft rejection, immunobiological techniques [32]. Another interesting situation is the heart transplantation in human immunodeficiency virus (HIV) infected cases [33]. This is still controversy [33-36]. Gupta et al. reported on a long-term follow-up of a heart transplant recipient with documented seroconversion to HIV-positive status 1 year after transplant and confirmed the high possibility for succeed in this practice [36].

Table 3. Some interesting reports on lung transplantation

Authors	Details
Sweet et al. [46]	Sweet et al. reported a study on lung transplantation and survival in children with cystic fibrosis [46]. Sweet et al. concluded that this procedure was still controversy [46].
Venkateswaran et al. [47]	Venkateswaran et al. reported that early donor management increased the retrieval rate of lungs for transplantation [47].
Liuo et al. [48]	Liuo et al. reported on lung transplantation and survival in children with cystic fibrosis [48]. Liuo et al. concluded that prolongation of life by lung transplantation could not be expected in children with cystic fibrosis [48].
Reams et al. [49]	Reams et al. reported on alemtuzumab in the treatment of refractory acute rejection and bronchiolitis obliterans syndrome after human lung transplantation [49].
Hachem et al. [50]	Hachem et al. reported on a randomized controlled trial of tacrolimus versus cyclosporine after lung transplantation [50]. Hachem et al. concluded that tacrolimus was associated with a lower burden of acute rejection and lymphocytic bronchitis than cyclosporine after lung transplantation [50].
Morton et al. [51]	Morton et al. reported on succeed in lung transplantation for adolescents in their setting [51].
Strüber et al. [52]	Strüber et al. reported on effects of exogenous surfactant instillation in clinical lung transplantation from a prospective, randomized trial [52]. Strüber et al. concluded that a protective effect of exogenous surfactant instillation to donor lungs before retrieval on post-lung transplantation surfactant function and on early clinical outcome could be determined [52].
Davenport et al. [53]	Davenport et al. reported on nrespiratory-related evoked potential elicited in tracheostomised lung transplant patients [53].
Bharat et al. [54]	Bharat et al. reported on the detection that CD4+25+ regulatory T cells limit Th1-autoimmunity by inducing IL-10 producing T cells following human lung transplantation [54].
Canales et al. [55]	Canales et al. reported on Predictors of chronic kidney disease in long-term survivors of lung and heart-lung transplantation [55].

B. Lung Transplantation

Heart transplantation is another organ transplantation at the early phase [44]. The beginning of lung transplantation rolls back to the 1940's when the Soviet Vladimir P. Demikhov performed the first lung transplants in animals [44]. Two decades later, James Hardy performed the first lung transplant in humans but it was failed [44]. Due to better surgery and medical technique at present, lung transplantation becomes easier and widely practiced for the patients with end stage lung diseases [45].

C. Kidney Transplantation

Kidney transplantation is another organ transplantation widely performed at present. This kind of transplantation has a long history for more than 40 years [56-58]. Kidney transplantation is indicated in end stage renal failure case. Indeed, the most present widely used means for treat the end stage renal failure is the dialysis. However, this does not bring curative outcome. Kidney transplantation is the new alternative with a lot of hope.

Table 4. Some interesting reports on kidney transplantation

Authors	Details
Lu et al. [59]	Lu et al. reported on kidney injury in transplantation-associated thrombotic microangiopathy [59].
Fontana et al. [60]	Fontana et al. reported on renal transplant compartment syndrome [60].
Catena et al. [61]	Catena et al. reported on gastrointestinal perforations following kidney transplantation [61].
Collura et al. [62]	Collura et al. reported on arterial changes in children undergoing renal transplantation [62].
Santangelo et al. [63]	Santangelo et al. reported on in situ elongation patch in right kidney transplantation [63].
Bertelli et al. [64]	Bertellie et al. studied on double kidney transplantation from multicenters [64]. Bertelli et al. concluded that double kidney transplantation was a safe approach for organ shortage [64].
Ferraresso et al. [65]	Ferraresso et al. reported on experience on kidney transplantation for childhood [65]. Ferraresso et al. concluded that long-term survivors of a kidney transplant received during childhood reached a high degree of rehabilitation despite a long period of immunosuppression [65].
Ilham et al. [66]	Ilham et al. reported on clinical significance of a positive flow crossmatch on the outcomes of cadaveric renal transplants [66]. Ilham et al. concluded that positive T-cell and B-cell FCXM transplant with a negative CDC-XM was associated with a higher incidence of rejection [66].

D. Liver Transplantation

Liver transplantation is another organ transplantation widely performed at present. Liver transplantation is indicated in end stage liver failure case. Liver transplantation is the new alternative with a lot of hope although the outcome is not favorable at present.

Table 5. Some interesting reports on liver transplantation

Authors	Details
Jiang et al. [67]	Jiang et al. reported on arcuate ligament syndrome inducing hepatic artery thrombosis after liver transplantation [67].
Jiang et al. [68]	Jiang et al. reported on effect of perioperative fluid therapy on early phase prognosis after liver transplantation [68].
Hori et al. [69]	Hori et al. reported on assessment of cardiac output in liver transplantation recipients [69].
Lu et al. [70]	Lu et al. reported on evaluation of the effect of lamivudine therapy preoperative to prevent hepatitis B virus recurrence after liver transplantation [70].
Yeh and Olthoff [71]	Yeh and Olthoff reported on live donor adult liver transplantation [71]. Yeh and Olthoff said that increasing the number of living-donor liver transplants would assist us to expedite transplant, prevent death, and possibly save more lives by expanding the criteria for transplant [71].
Moya Herráiz et al. [72]	Moya Herráiz et al. reported on liver transplantation in patients with benign hepatic lesions [72].
Perkins [73]	Perkins et al. reported on sinusoidal obstructive syndrome, which was a rare and stressful indication for liver transplantation [73].
Rossi et al. [74]	Rossi et al. reported on combined liver-kidney transplantation in polycystic disease [74].

After Transplantation

After transplantation, the patient should be closed monitored. The opportunistic infection due to the immunosuppresive status of the patients receiving immunosuppressive drug administration should be focused. The survival rates of different kinds of transplantation are different. This cannot be easily expected. in addition to physical status, psychological aspect of the patient after transplantation needs concern. Psychological support is needed. The family approach to verify if the patient has good quality of life within the family after transplantation is recommended and very helpful. The cause of death for any cases after transplantation might be due to graft rejection. However, this is usually controllable by the use of good immunosuppressive drug. The other condition to be mentioned is graft versus host (GVD) [75-77]. GVD is a serious condition and should be carefully managed. Early sign as skin manifestation can be observed [75-77]. If GVD is suspected, prompt treatment with daclizumab and intravenous corticosteroids should be given and the patient might survive without evidence of systemic GVH [78].

References

[1] Okabayashi K, Asashima M. Regenerative medicine: history and perspectives. *Nippon Rinsho*. 2008 May;66(5):825-30.

[2] Roth CA, Lenfant C. Implants, transplants, and other parts of the medicine of the future. *Ann Biomed Eng*. 1990;18(4):337-46.

[3] Lee S. Historical significance on rat organ transplantation. *Microsurgery*. 1990;11(2):115-21.

[4] Agthong S, Wiwanitkit V. Cadaver donation: a retrospective review at the King Chulalongkorn Memorial Hospital, Bangkok. *Southeast Asian J Trop Med Public Health*. 2002;33 Suppl 3:166-7.

[5] Wiwanitkit V, Agthong S. The rate of anti-HIV seropositivity among donated cadavers: experience in a cadaver donation center. *Viral Immunol*. 2002;15(4):659-60.

[6] Len O, Pahissa A. Donor-transmitted infections. *Enferm Infecc Microbiol Clin*. 2007 Mar;25(3):204-12.

[7] Centers for Disease Control and Prevention (CDC). Transplantation-transmitted tuberculosis--Oklahoma and Texas, 2007. *MMWR Morb Mortal Wkly Rep*. 2008 Apr 4;57(13):333-6.

[8] Hassan SS, Wilhelmus KR, Dahl P, Davis GC, Roberts RT, Ross KW, Varnum BH; Medical Review Subcommittee of the Eye Bank Association of America. Infectious disease risk factors of corneal graft donors. *Arch Ophthalmol*. 2008 Feb;126(2):235-9.

[9] Palacios G, Druce J, Du L, Tran T, Birch C, Briese T, Conlan S, Quan PL, Hui J, Marshall J, Simons JF, Egholm M, Paddock CD, Shieh WJ, Goldsmith CS, Zaki SR, Catton M, Lipkin WI. A new arenavirus in a cluster of fatal transplant-associated diseases. *N Engl J Med*. 2008 Mar 6;358(10):991-8.

[10] Gajewska M, Wielgos M, Kamiński P, Marianowski P, Malejczyk M, Majewski S, Marianowski L. The occurrence of genital types of human papillomavirus in normal pregnancy and in pregnant renal transplant recipients. *Neuro Endocrinol Lett*. 2006 Aug;27(4):529-34.

[11] Kumar D, Humar A. Pandemic influenza and its implications for transplantation. *Am J Transplant*. 2006 Jul;6(7):1512-7.

[12] Zöllner B, Feucht HH, Sterneck M, Schäfer H, Rogiers X, Fischer L. Clinical reactivation after liver transplantation with an unusual minor strain of hepatitis B virus in an occult carrier. *Liver Transpl*. 2006 Aug;12(8):1283-9.

[13] Campos S, Caramori M, Teixeira R, Afonso J Jr, Carraro R, Strabelli T, Samano M, Pêgo-Fernandes P, Jatene F. Bacterial and fungal pneumonias after lung transplantation.*Transplant Proc*. 2008 Apr;40(3):822-4.

[14] Chrastina N, Zilinska Z, Breza J Jr, Breza J. CMV infection and CMV disease in kidney transplant recipients--our experience. *Bratisl Lek Listy*. 2008;109(1):42.

[15] Mattner F, Sykora KW, Meissner B, Heim A. An adenovirus type F41 outbreak in a pediatric bone marrow transplant unit: analysis of clinical impact and preventive strategies. *Pediatr Infect Dis J*. 2008 May;27(5):419-24.

[16] Nordquist BC, Aronson LR. Pyogranulomatous cystitis associated with Toxoplasma gondii infection in a cat after renal transplantation. *J Am Vet Med Assoc*. 2008 Apr 1;232(7):1010-2.

[17] Alkhunaizi AM, Al-Tawfiq JA, Al-Shawaf MH. Transfusion-transmitted malaria in a kidney transplant recipient. How safe is our blood transfusion? *Saudi Med J.* 2008 Feb;29(2):293-5.

[18] Schmoldt S, Schuhegger R, Wendler T, Huber I, Söllner H, Hogardt M, Arbogast H, Heesemann J, Bader L, Sing A. Molecular evidence of nosocomial Pneumocystis jirovecii transmission among 16 patients after kidney transplantation. *J Clin Microbiol.* 2008 Mar;46(3):966-71.

[19] Yilmaz A, Hazar V, Akçam M, Inanç-Gürer E, Ceken K, Artan R. Burkitt's lymphoma following a pediatric liver transplantation: predictive negative value of serologic response to Epstein-Barr virus. *Turk J Pediatr.* 2007 Oct-Dec;49(4):434-6.

[20] Waldman M, Kopp JB. Parvovirus-B19-associated complications in renal transplant recipients. *Nat Clin Pract Nephrol.* 2007 Oct;3(10):540-50

[21] Safdar A, Papadopoulos EB, Young JW. Breakthrough Scedosporium apiospermum (Pseudallescheria boydii) brain abscess during therapy for invasive pulmonary aspergillosis following high-risk allogeneic hematopoietic stem cell transplantation. Scedosporiasis and recent advances in antifungal therapy. *Transpl Infect Dis* 2002;4:212-7

[22] Injured Thai pop star taken off respirator, moved from intensive care. Utusan (2003, December 9) Available at Http:// http://health.surfwax.com/files/Abscesses.html.

[23] Nesky MA, McDougal EC, Peacock Jr JE. Pseudallescheria boydii brain abscess successfully treated with voriconazole and surgical drainage: case report and literature review of central nervous system pseudallescheriasis.

[24] Hachimi-Idrissi S, Willemsen M, Desprechins B, Naessens A, Goossens A, De Meirleir L, Ramet J. Pseudallescheria boydii and brain abscesses. *Pediatr Infect Dis J* 1990;9:737-41

[25] Little AM. An overview of HLA typing for hematopoietic stem cell transplantation. *Methods Mol Med.* 2007;134:35-49.

[26] Hurley CK, Wade JA, Oudshoorn M, Middleton D, Kukuruga D, Navarrete C, Christiansen F, Hegland J, Ren EC, Andersen I, Cleaver SA, Brautbar C, Raffoux C. A special report: histocompatibility testing guidelines for hematopoietic stem cell transplantation using volunteer donors. Quality Assurance and Donor Registries Working Groups of the World Marrow Donor Association. *Hum Immunol.* 1999 Apr;60(4):347-60.

[27] Gergely M. The first heart transplantation. *Orv Hetil.* 1992 Mar 29;133(13):817-9.

[28] Lansman SL, Ergin MA, Griepp RB. The history of heart and heart-lung transplantation. *Cardiovasc Clin.* 1990;20(2):3-19.

[29] Dark JH. History of heart-lung transplantation. *Lung.* 1990;168 Suppl:1165-8.

[30] Mendeloff EN. The history of pediatric heart and lung transplantation. *Pediatr Transplant.* 2002 Aug;6(4):270-9.

[31] DiBardino DJ. The history and development of cardiac transplantation. *Tex Heart Inst J.* 1999;26(3):198-205.

[32] Karpawich PP. Pediatric cardiac resynchronization pacing therapy. *Curr Opin Cardiol.* 2007 Mar;22(2):72-6.

[33] Law YM. Pathophysiology and diagnosis of allograft rejection in pediatric heart transplantation. *Curr Opin Cardiol.* 2007 Mar;22(2):66-71.

[34] Jahangiri B, Haddad H. Cardiac transplantation in HIV-positive patients: are we there yet? *J Heart Lung Transplant.* 2007 Feb;26(2):103-7.

[35] Stock PG, Roland ME. Evolving clinical strategies for transplantation in the HIV-positive recipient. *Transplantation.* 2007 Sep 15;84(5):563-71.

[36] Gupta S, Markham DW, Mammen PP, Kaiser P, Patel P, Ring WS, Drazner MH. Long-term follow-up of a heart transplant recipient with documented seroconversion to HIV-positive status 1 year after transplant. *Am J Transplant.* 2008 Apr;8(4):893-6.

[37] Lehmkuhl H, Hummel M, Kobashigawa J, Ladenburger S, Rothenburger M, Sack F, Dengler T, Hetzer R. Enteric-coated mycophenolate-sodium in heart transplantation: efficacy, safety, and pharmacokinetic compared with mycophenolate mofetil. *Transplant Proc.* 2008 May;40(4):953-5.

[38] Quarta CC, Potena L, Grigioni F, Scalone A, Magnani G, Coccolo F, Fallani F, Russo A, Branzi A. Safety and efficacy of ezetimibe with low doses of simvastatin in heart transplant recipients. *J Heart Lung Transplant.* 2008 Jun;27(6):685-8.

[39] Potena L, Grigioni F, Masetti M, Magnani G, Coccolo F, Fallani F, Russo A, Pizzuti M, Scalone A, Bianchi IG, Branzi A. Long-term effect of folic acid therapy in heart transplant recipients: follow-up analysis of a randomized study. *Transplantation.* 2008 Apr 27;85(8):1146-50.

[40] Singh H, Merry AF, Ruygrok P, Ruttley A. Treatment of recurrent chest pain in a heart transplant recipient using spinal cord stimulation. *Anaesth Intensive Care.* 2008 Mar;36(2):242-4.

[41] Letsas KP, Weber R, Arentz T, Kalusche D. Catheter ablation of recipient-to-donor atrioatrial conduction with wenckebach-like phenomenon after orthotopic heart transplantation. *J Heart Lung Transplant.* 2008 Aug;27(8):917-20

[42] Lacy MQ, Dispenzieri A, Hayman SR, Kumar S, Kyle RA, Rajkumar SV, Edwards BS, Rodeheffer RJ, Frantz RP, Kushwaha SS, Clavell AL, Dearani JA, Sundt TM, Daly RC, McGregor CG, Gastineau DA, Litzow MR, Gertz MA. Autologous stem cell transplant after heart transplant for light chain (Al) amyloid cardiomyopathy. *J Heart Lung Transplant.* 2008 Aug;27(8):823-9.

[43] Marelli D, Kobashigawa J, Hamilton MA, Moriguchi JD, Kermani R, Ardehali A, Patel J, Noguchi E, Beygui R, Laks H, Plunkett M, Shemin R, Esmailian F. Long-term outcomes of heart transplantation in older recipients. *J Heart Lung Transplant.* 2008 Aug;27(8):830-4.

[44] García-Covarrubias L, Salerno TA, Panos AL, Pham SM. Lung transplantation. State of the art. *Gac Med Mex.* 2007 Jul-Aug;143(4):323-32.

[45] Trindade AJ, Palmer SM. Current concepts and controversies in lung transplantation. *Respir Care Clin N Am.* 2004 Dec;10(4):427-47, v.

[46] Sweet SC, Aurora P, Benden C, Wong JY, Goldfarb SB, Elidemir O, Woo MS, Mallory GB Jr; International Pediatric Lung Transplant Collaborative. Lung transplantation and survival in children with cystic fibrosis: solid statistics--flawed interpretation. *Pediatr Transplant.* 2008 Mar;12(2):129-36.

[47] Venkateswaran RV, Patchell VB, Wilson IC, Mascaro JG, Thompson RD, Quinn DW, Stockley RA, Coote JH, Bonser RS. Early donor management increases the retrieval rate of lungs for transplantation. *Ann Thorac Surg*. 2008 Jan;85(1):278-86

[48] Liou TG, Adler FR, Cox DR, Cahill BC. Lung transplantation and survival in children with cystic fibrosis. *N Engl J Med*. 2007 Nov 22;357(21):2143-52.

[49] Reams BD, Musselwhite LW, Zaas DW, Steele MP, Garantziotis S, Eu PC, Snyder LD, Curl J, Lin SS, Davis RD, Palmer SM. Alemtuzumab in the treatment of refractory acute rejection and bronchiolitis obliterans syndrome after human lung transplantation. *Am J Transplant*. 2007 Dec;7(12):2802-8.

[50] Hachem RR, Yusen RD, Chakinala MM, Meyers BF, Lynch JP, Aloush AA, Patterson GA, Trulock EP. A randomized controlled trial of tacrolimus versus cyclosporine after lung transplantation. *J Heart Lung Transplant*. 2007 Oct;26(10):1012-8.

[51] Morton JM, Malouf MA, Plit ML, Spratt PM, Glanville AR. Successful lung transplantation for adolescents at a hospital for adults. *Med J Aust*. 2007 Sep 3;187(5):278-82.

[52] Strüber M, Fischer S, Niedermeyer J, Warnecke G, Gohrbandt B, Görler A, Simon AR, Haverich A, Hohlfeld JM. Effects of exogenous surfactant instillation in clinical lung transplantation: a prospective, randomized trial. *J Thorac Cardiovasc Surg*. 2007 Jun;133(6):1620-5.

[53] Davenport PW, Martin AD, Chou YL, Alexander-Miller S. Respiratory-related evoked potential elicited in tracheostomised lung transplant patients. *Eur Respir J*. 2006 Aug;28(2):391-6.

[54] Bharat A, Fields RC, Steward N, Trulock EP, Patterson GA, Mohanakumar T. CD4+25+ regulatory T cells limit Th1-autoimmunity by inducing IL-10 producing T cells following human lung transplantation. *Am J Transplant*. 2006 Aug;6(8):1799-808.

[55] Canales M, Youssef P, Spong R, Ishani A, Savik K, Hertz M, Ibrahim HN. Predictors of chronic kidney disease in long-term survivors of lung and heart-lung transplantation. *Am J Transplant*. 2006 Sep;6(9):2157-63.

[56] Brower PA, Harrison JH, Landes RR. Renal transplantation: history. *Urology*. 1977 Jul;10(1 Suppl):5-10.

[57] Merrill JP. A historical perspective of renal transplantation. *Proc Clin Dial Transplant Forum*. 1979;9:221-5.

[58] Artifact: the first kidney transplanter (Dr. Emerich Ullmann). *Med Instrum*. 1974 May-Jun;8(3):193.

[59] Lu M, Zou WZ, Zhang Y, Wang SL, Wang W. Kidney injury in transplantation-associated thrombotic microangiopathy. *Beijing Da Xue Xue Bao*. 2008 Aug 18;40(4):392-4.

[60] Fontana I, Bertocchi M, Centanaro M, Diviacco P, De Negri A, Ghinolfi D, Tommasi G, Magoni Rossi A, Santori G, Dallatomasina S, Nardi I, Piaggio F, Moraglia E, Valente U. Renal transplant compartment syndrome: a case report. *Transplant Proc*. 2008 Jul-Aug;40(6):2065-6.

[61] Catena F, Ansaloni L, Gazzotti F, Bertelli R, Severi S, Coccolini F, Fuga G, Nardo B, D'Alessandro L, Faenza A, Pinna AD. Gastrointestinal perforations following kidney transplantation. *Transplant Proc*. 2008 Jul-Aug;40(6):1895-6.

[62] Collura G, Capozza N, Francalanci P, Caione P. Arterial changes in children undergoing renal transplantation. *Transplant Proc*. 2008 Jul-Aug;40(6):1891-4.

[63] Santangelo M, Spinosa G, Grassia S, Clemente M, Caggiano M, Pelosio L, Scotti A, Tammaro V, Nappi R, Di Capua F, Renda A. In situ elongation patch in right kidney transplantation. *Transplant Proc*. 2008 Jul-Aug;40(6):1871-2.

[64] Bertelli R, Nardo B, Capocasale E, Cappelli G, Cavallari G, Mazzoni MP, Benozzi L, Dalla Valle R, Fuga G, Busi N, Gilioli C, Albertazzi A, Stefoni S, Pinna AD, Faenza A. Multicenter study on double kidney transplantation. *Transplant Proc*. 2008 Jul-Aug;40(6):1869-70.

[65] Ferraresso M, Ghio L, Raiteri M, Belingheri M, Beretta C, Martina V, Edefonti A, Berardinelli L. Pediatric kidney transplantation: a snapshot 10 years later. *Transplant Proc*. 2008 Jul-Aug;40(6):1852-3.

[66] Ilham MA, Winkler S, Coates E, Rizzello A, Rees TJ, Asderakis A. Clinical significance of a positive flow crossmatch on the outcomes of cadaveric renal transplants. *Transplant Proc*. 2008 Jul-Aug;40(6):1839-43.

[67] Jiang ZJ, Liang TB, Feng XN, Wang WL, Shen Y, Zhang M, Wu J, Xu X, Zheng SS. Arcuate ligament syndrome inducing hepatic artery thrombosis after liver transplantation. *Hepatobiliary Pancreat Dis Int*. 2008 Aug;7(4):433-6.

[68] Jiang GQ, Peng MH, Yang DH. Effect of perioperative fluid therapy on early phase prognosis after liver transplantation. *Hepatobiliary Pancreat Dis Int*. 2008 Aug;7(4):367-72.

[69] Hori T, Yamamoto C, Yagi S, Iida T, Taniguchi K, Hasegawa T, Yamakado K, Hori Y, Takeda K, Maruyama K, Uemoto S. Assessment of cardiac output in liver transplantation recipients. *Hepatobiliary Pancreat Dis Int*. 2008 Aug;7(4):362-6.

[70] Lu AW, Zheng SS, Wu MP, Shen Y, Yang RW. Reevaluation of the effect of lamivudine therapy preoperative to prevent HBV recurrence after liver transplantation. Hepatobiliary *Pancreat Dis Int*. 2008 Aug;7(4):357-61.

[71] Yeh H, Olthoff KM. Live donor adult liver transplantation. *Curr Opin Organ Transplant*. 2008 Jun;13(3):241-6.

[72] Moya Herráiz A, Torres-Quevedo R, Mir Pallardó J. Liver transplantation in patients with benign hepatic lesions. *Cir Esp*. 2008 Aug;84(2):60-6.

[73] Perkins JD. Sinusoidal obstructive syndrome: a rare and stressful indication for liver transplantation. *Liver Transpl*. 2008 Aug;14(8):1219-20.

[74] Rossi M, Spoletini G, Bussotti A, Lai Q, Travaglia D, Ferretti S, Poli L, Ginanni Corradini S, Merli M, Novelli G, Mennini G, Pugliese F, Berloco PB. Combined liver-kidney transplantation in polycystic disease: case reports. *Transplant Proc*. 2008 Jul-Aug;40(6):2075-6.

[75] Imanguli MM, Alevizos I, Brown R, Pavletic SZ, Atkinson JC. Oral graft-versus-host disease. *Oral Dis*. 2008 Jul;14(5):396-412.

[76] Martin PJ, Carpenter PA, Sanders JE, Flowers ME. Diagnosis and clinical management of chronic graft-versus-host disease. *Int J Hematol.* 2004 Apr;79(3):221-8

[77] Akpek G. Clinical grading in chronic graft-versus-host disease: is it time for change? *Leuk Lymphoma.* 2002 Jun;43(6):1211-20.

[78] Yashar S, Wu SS, Binder SW, Cotliar J. Acute graft-versus-host disease after pediatric solid organ transplant. *J Drugs Dermatol.* 2008 May;7(5):467-9.

Chapter VI

ADVENT IN RADIOTHERAPY, RADIOINTERVENTION AND RADIOSURGERY

INTRODUCTION TO RADIOLOGY

Radioactive substance is classified as a new group of elements that human beings knew for about 1 century. After the discovery of Curie Family [1-4], radioactive substance becomes on focused interested of global scientist. There are many researches on radioactive substance. Application of radioactive substance for usage is continuously proposed. At present, radioactive substances can be used in industry as well as medicine. The main focus of radioactive use in medicine is for treatment of tumor. Also it is applied for diagnosis as radioassay.

Parallel to radioactive substance, rays are also focused for its application in medicine. After the discovery of X-ray [5-8], the application in medicine is a big jump of medical world. With use of X-ray, physician can visualize the internal structure of human being and used it for diagnosis. This is the history of development of a famous medical science, radiology. At present, radiology is a necessary medical science that helps both diagnose and treat of patients. Radiology unit is a basic unit for all hospital. Basically, three basic main branches of radiology are described as radiodiagnosis, radiotherapy and nuclear medicine. Radiodiagnosis focuses mainly on diagnosis of disorders by usage of several means of imaging technology in medicine. Radiotherapy focuses mainly on treatment and will be mainly detailed and discussed in this chapter. Finally, nuclear medicine focuses mainly on both diagnosis and treatment based on usage of radioactive substances. Important details of nuclear medicine based treatment will also be detailed and discussed in this chapter.

Table 1. Three basic radioactive emitted rays

Rays	Details
alpha ray	It is proved to be the nucleus of Helium and has mass about 4 U. Its electrical power is equal to + 2e and has power equal to 4 MeV. It has low penetrating activity.
beta ray	Its electrical property is equal to -1e and has mass about electron. The power is equal to 0.025 - 3.5 MeV.
gamma ray	It is electrical neutral and accepted as an electromagnetic wave. The power is equal to 0.04 - 3.2 MeV and has the strongest penetrating power comparing to other two previously mentioned rays.

RADIOTHERAPY

Radiotherapy is a specific application of radiology for treatment of disorder. This focuses mainly on application or rays and radioactive substances for treatment. To applied radiotherapy to patients, there can be three common practices:

a) Classical Radiotherapy

This makes used of rays, which are mainly X-ray and gamma ray emitted from Cobalt 60, for treatment of disorders. This is broadly used in present medicine. Several cancers are subjected to be treated with radiotherapy. For example, nasopharyngeal carcinoma, an Ebstien-Barr virus related cancer, is subjected to treat by classical radiotherapy or irradiation. Radiotherapy can be used alone or as combination or adjuvant to other therapy such as chemotherapy. Some important aspects on classical radiotherapy for several important cancers will be herby presented in Table 2.

It should be noted that the important complications of classical radiotherapy is the destructive of nearby non-defected part of the patients. This usually makes suffering to the patients and prevents the good correspondence to the classical radiotherapy treatment. Taking special care to the nearby tissue for the patients receiving the classical radiotherapy is therefore an important supportive and symptomatic treatment issue for this group of patients.

b) Brachytherapy

Brachytherapy is another common mode of radiothreapy. This makes use of radioactive element insertion or implantation next to the tumor. It bases on the fact that radioactive element will emit rays that can treat or kill the uncontrolled growth parts of tumor. The most famous usage of brachytherapy is for treatment of cervical cancer. Some important reports on brachytherapy will be presented in Table 3.

Table 2. Important reports on cancer treatment by classical radiotherapy

Authors	Details
Braendengen et al. [9]	Braendengen et al. reported on randomized phase III study comparing preoperative radiotherapy with chemoradiotherapy in nonresectable rectal cancer [9]. Braendengen et al. concluded that chemoradiotherapy improved local control, time to treatment failure, and cancer-specific survival compared with radiotherapy alone in patients with nonresectable rectal cancer [9].
Constantine et al. [10]	Constantine et al. reported on feasibility of accelerated whole-breast radiation in the treatment of patients with ductal carcinoma in situ of the breast [10]. Constantine et al. demonstrated the feasibility of treating the whole breast for ductal carcinoma in situ with a hypofractionated regimen, with modest acute and late toxicity in this paper [10].
Tsubokura et al. [11]	Tsubokura et al. reported on radiotherapy hypofractionation in early breast cancer [11].
Ganswindt et al. [12]	Ganswindt et al. reported on adjuvant radiotherapy for patients with locally advanced prostate cancer [12]. Ganswindt et al. said that this modality resulted in significant improved biochemical progression-free survival and local control [12].
Berk [13]	Berk reported on radiation therapy as primary and adjuvant treatment for local and regional melanoma [13]
Sanfilippo et al. [14]	Sanfilippo et al. reported on phase I/II study of biweekly paclitaxel and radiation in androgen-ablated locally advanced prostate cancer. [14].
Mufazalov et al. [15]	Mufazalov et al. reported on radiotherapy of malignant brain gliomas using teniposide [15].
Hughes et al. [16]	Hughes et al. published on the safety study of induction chemotherapy followed by synchronous radiotherapy and cetuximab in stage III non-small cell lung cancer [16].
Naito et al. [17]	Naito et al. reported on concurrent chemoradiotherapy with cisplatin and vinorelbine for stage III non-small cell lung cancer [17].
Ku and Ilson [18]	Ku and Ilson reported on preoperative therapy in esophageal cancer [18].
Tsoutsou et al. [19]	Tsoutsou et al. reported on hypofractionated /accelerated radiotherapy with cytoprotection combined with vinorelbine and liposomal doxorubicin for locally advanced non-small cell lung cancer [19].
Borone et al. [20]	Borone et al. reported on induction chemotherapy followed by concurrent chemoradiotherapy in advanced head and neck squamous cell carcinoma [20].
Yokoyama et al. [21]	Yokoyama et al. reported on a phase II multicenter trial of concurrent chemoradiotherapy with weekly nedaplatin in advanced uterine cervical carcinoma [21]
FitzGerald et al. [22]	FitzGerald et al. reported on processes for quality improvements in radiation oncology clinical trials [22].
Brizel et al. [23]	Brizel et al. reported on Phase II study of palifermin and concurrent chemoradiation in head and neck squamous cell carcinoma [23].
Socinski et al. [24]	Socinski et al. reported on randomized phase II trial of induction chemotherapy followed by concurrent chemotherapy and dose-escalated thoracic conformal radiotherapy in stage III non-small-cell lung cancer [24].
de Vreeze et al. [25]	de Vreeze et al. reported that effectiveness of radiotherapy in myxoid sarcomas was associated with a dense vascular pattern [25].

Table 3. Important reports on brachytherapy

Authors	Details
Janaki et al. [26]	Janaki et al. reported on epidural analgesia during brachytherapy for cervical cancer patients [26].
Papagelopoulos et al. [27]	Papagelopoulos et al. reported on free vascularised tissue transfer and brachytherapy for soft-tissue sarcomas of the extremities [27].
Sedda et al. [28]	Sedda et al. reported on dermatological high-dose-rate brachytherapy for the treatment of basal and squamous cell carcinoma [28].
Miura et al. [29]	Miura et al. reported on radiation pneumonitis caused by a migrated brachytherapy seed lodged in the lung [29].
Potter et al. [30]	Potter et al. discussed on present status and future of high-precision image guided adaptive brachytherapy for cervix carcinoma [30]. Potter et al. noted that this technique provided a very high local control rate with minor treatment related morbidity [30].
Raisali et al. [31]	Raisali et al. reported on Monte Carlo and experimental characterization of the first AMIRS (103)Pd brachytherapy source [31].
Roessler et al. [32]	Roessler et al. reported on naesthesia for brachytherapy [32]. Roessler et al. noted that anaesthesiologists played an important role in the ongoing challenge to provide safe and pain-free conditions for an optimum brachytherapy treatment effect [32].
Engle et al. [33]	Engle et al. reported on effect of laparoscopic guidance on gynecologic interstitial brachytherapy [33].
Mehdizadeh et al. [34]	Mehdizadeh et al. reported on a lpha particle vascular brachytherapy in the treatment of in-stent Restenosis [34].
Semrau et al. [35]	Semrau et al. reported on successful treatment of field cancerization of the scalp by surface mould brachytherapy [35].
Wojcik et al. [36]	Wojcik et al. reported on enhanced level of micronuclei in peripheral blood lymphocytes of patients treated for restenosis with (32)P endovascular brachytherapy [33].However, Wojcik et al. noted that although brachytherapy of restenosis with (32)P led to weak enhancement of the micronucleus frequency in lymphocytes, the effect was not seen in all patients [36].
Fabrini et al. [37]	Fabrini et al. reported on high-dose-rate brachytherapy in a large squamous cell carcinoma of the hand [37].
Julow et al. [38]	Julow et al. reported on prediction of volumetric change in the "triple ring" caused by glioma I-125 brachytherapy [38].
Ritter [39]	Ritter reported on body mass index and prostate-specific antigen failure following brachytherapy for localized prostate cancer [39].

Similar to classical radiotherapy, destructive of nearby non-defected part of the patients also brings suffering to the patients and prevents the good correspondence to the brachytherapy. Supportive and symptomatic treatment issue for this group of patients are also necessary.

c) Radioactive Substance Ingestion

This is specifically used in nuclear medicine for treatment of thyroid disorder. Specific radioactive element, Iodine 131, which has the half life equal to 8 days, is used. This topic is well described in thyroidology. This application is used mainly for any hyperthyroidism cases that are not response to basic medical therapy. Some important reports on radioactive substance ingestion for treatment will be listed in Table 4.

Table 4. Some important reports on radioactive substance ingestion for treatment

Authors	Details
Zhao et al. [40]	Zhao et al. reported on Inhibitory effects of immunotargeting of Chinese cobra cytotoxin and iodine-131 against nasopharyngeal carcinoma cells in vitro [40].
Sanyal et al. [41]	Sanyal et al. reported on use of methotrexate to treat isolated Graves ophthalmopathy developing years after thyroidectomy and iodine 131 treatment of papillary thyroid cancer [41].
Garsi et al. [42]	Garsi et al. reported on therapeutic administration of 131I for differentiated thyroid cancer [42].
Rajendran et al. [43]	Rajendran et al. reported on myeloablative 131I-tositumomab radioimmunotherapy in treating non-Hodgkin's lymphoma [43]. Rajendran et al. concluded that dosimetry based on whole-body retention might underestimate the organ doses, and a preferable approach was to assess organ-specific doses by accounting for actual radionuclide biodistribution [43].
Mäenpää et al. [44]	Mäenpää et al. reported that 3700 MBq activity was note more effective for ablation of the thyroid remnant than 1100 MBq activity amd the 3700 MBq activity was also associated with more adverse effects [44]
Schaefer-Cutillo and Friedberg [45]	Schaefer-Cutillo and Friedberg reported on non-myeloablative radioimmunotherapy based on Iodine 131-tositumomab and ibritumomab tiuxetan, radioimmunoconjugates targeting the CD20 antigen for non-Hodgkin's lymphoma [45].
Lau and Lai [46]	Lau and Lai reported on treatment of unresectable hepatocellular carcinoma with transarterial radioembolization using iodine-131-lipiodol [46].
Kim et al. [47]	Kim et al. reported for limited cytoprotective effects of amifostine in high-dose radioactive iodine 131-treated well-differentiated thyroid cancer patients [47].
de Kraker et al. [48]	de Kraker et al. reported on Iodine-131-metaiodobenzylguanidine as initial induction therapy in stage 4 neuroblastoma patients over 1 year of age [48].
Nwosu et al. [49]	Nwosu et al. reported on results from assessment of the efficacy and toxicity of (131)I-metaiodobenzylguanidine therapy for metastatic neuroendocrine tumors [49]. Nwosu et al. concluded that (131)I- metaiodobenzylguanidine could improve symptoms in more than half of the patients with metastatic neuroendocrine tumours and survival was increased in those patients who reported a symptomatic response to therapy [49].

RADIOINTERVENTION

Radiointervention is a new applied radiology. It should be noted that the access to some specific parts of human body seems difficult such as intra-arterial or intravenous sites. If there is a specific problem or pathology related to these structures, it will be hard to treat. However, with the concept of radiointervention, the treatment could be feasible. Intervention makes use of probing to small hard-to-reach site. This can be applied in many aspects such as vascular surgery. There are many good examples of radiointervention such as embolectomy. Embolectomy is the best example because it directly deals with the small portions within the vessels. Important reports on application of radiointervention for treatment of hard-to-treat condition are shown in Table 5.

Table 5. Examples of application of radiointervention for treatment in medicine

Authors	Details
Jarabek et al. [50]	Jarabek et al. reported on results of therapy of lower extremity ischemic disease by angiosurgery and radiointervention methods [50].
Black et al. [51]	Black et al. reported on contemporary results of angioplasty-based infrainguinal percutaneous interventions [51].
Kuo et al. [52]	Kuo et al. reported on catheter-directed embolectomy, fragmentation, and thrombolysis for the treatment of massive pulmonary embolism after failure of systemic thrombolysis [52].
Valpreda et al. [53]	Valpreda et al. reported on stenting of transplant renal artery stenosis [53].
Giller et al. [54]	Giller et al. discussed on multidisciplinary treatment of a large cerebral dural arteriovenous fistula using embolization, surgery, and radiosurgery [54].
Lee et al. [55]	Lee et al. reported on long-term outcomes of endoluminal therapy for chronic atherosclerotic occlusive mesenteric disease [55].
Mansour et al. [56]	Mansour et al. reported on adiological central vein treatment in vascular access [56].
Wang et al. [57]	Wang et al. reported on endovascular treatment of giant intracranial aneurysms with willis covered stents [57].

An interesting topic of radiointervention is that not any physician can perform this procedure because it is hard and can pose a serious complication. Specific training course is needed. As previously mentioned, the radiointervention procedure is usually for vascular approach, therefore, this kind of treatment requires closed monitoring in specific ward. An operative room with anesthetic function is needed. Briefly, the radiointervention procedure starts with radiodiagnosis of problematic site with help of radiodiagnosis technique. After getting the target, planning for appropriate approach is needed. The planning usually makes use of basic knowledge on vascular anatomy of human beings. The most proper track for approaching will be selected. Then it reaches the most important step, the real instrument insertion or intervention. Insertion of interventive tool into the vascular canal must be gently done. Closed monitoring during this process is required. Leakage can be possible at any second and requires prompt correction if occurs. When the tool reaches the targeted site, the final active (either embolization, removal, dilation or injection) will be done. Monitoring of completeness of mission is necessary before removing out of the tool from the vascular canal. Wound closing at the removal site is the latest step. Ward admitting for closed monitoring after operation is suggested. Observation of bleeding at wound is needed. Also, observation on the patients' general condition as well as the possible complication is required. These post operative managements should be set for at least one day period.

Table 6. Some important publications on radiosurgery

Authors	Details
Gerszten et al. [58]	Gerszten et al. reported a study on radiosurgery for benign intradural spinal tumors [58]. Gerszten et al. found that single fraction radiosurgery was detected to be clinically effective for the treatment of benign extramedullary spinal neoplasms [58].
Mathieu et al. [59]	Mathieu et al. reported on tumor bed radiosurgery after resection of cerebral metastases [59]. Fuller et al. reported on virtual HDR CyberKnife treatment for localized prostatic carcinoma [60]. Fuller et al. found that constructing CyberKnife stereotactic body radiotherapy plans that closely recapitulated HDR dosimetry and delivered the plans noninvasively was feasible [60].
Kondziolka et al. [61]	Kondziolka et al. reported radiosurgery as definitive management of intracranial meningiomas [61]. Kondziolka et al. concluded that Stereotactic radiosurgery provided high rates of tumor growth control or regression in patients with benign meningiomas with low risk [61].
Ryu et al. [62]	Ryu et al. reported on pain control by image-guided radiosurgery for solitary spinal metastasis [62].
Franzin et al. [63]	Franzin et al. reported on neuroophthalmological evaluation after gamma knife surgery for cavernous sinus meningiomas [63]. Franzin et al. concluded that gamma knife surgery was a safe and effective treatment for tumors located close to the optic pathways [63].
Lekovic et al. [64]	Lekovic et al. reported that excellent control of pineal region brain tumors could be derived with gamma knife surgery when it was applied in conjunction with surgery, conventional radiation therapy, or both [64].
Romanelli et al. [65]	Romanelli et al. reported on multicenter trial on CyberKnife surgery [65]. Romanell et al. concluded that CyberKnife brought high conformality and submillimetric accuracy of frame-based systems combined with the possibility of delivering radiation in several sessions [65].
Li et al. [66]	Li et al. reported on CyberKnife rhizotomy for facetogenic back pain [66]
Pusztaszeri et al. [67]	Pusztaszeri et al. reported on radiosurgery for trigeminal neuralgia using a linear accelerator with BrainLab system [67].
Taschner et al. [68]	Taschner et al. reported on gamma knife surgery for arteriovenous malformations in the brain [68].

RADIOSURGERY

Radiosurgery is the modern application of radiology. In the past, surgery was based on knife and other invasive tools. This was performed in limited specific operative room and requires complete team for surgery. Also, it usually took time for each surgical procedure and post operative following up. The smallest wound with the least pain is the present aim of surgery. To reach this aim, there are several alternatives to classical surgery. Radiosurgery is an alternative that helps physician to reach this concept. Radiosurgery makes use of ray for surgical procedure. It can be said that ray is used as a knife. There are many new reports on radiosurgery. A gamma knife is one of the most well-known radiosurgical tools. This is very useful for neurosurgery. Surgical procedure for deep brain lesion is usually hard and brings several complications; however, this can be controlled by radiosurgery. It can be easy thing with help of gamma knife. The procedures cause small wounds, required short period of surgical procedure and does not need long term post operative care. In addition, the complication is not high. There are also other applications on radiosurgery. The author hereby will present some important published works on this topic (Table 6).

An interesting aspect of this specific new technique, radiosurgery, is the feasibility to use. This technique is considered expensive although it is highly effective. Cost effectiveness of this technique of surgery might prevent some patients to reach. This can prevent its usefulness. However, Cho et al. studied on socioeconomic costs of open surgery and gamma knife radiosurgery for benign cranial base tumors and reported that Gamma knife radiosurgery was an acceptable treatment the our patients because it reduced hospital stays and workdays lost and decreased complications, mortality, socioeconomic loss, and achieve better cost-effectiveness [69]. In addition, the affordability of different patients to this technique differs. This can be a big barrier for equilibrium for treatment assessment of all patients. How to cope with this problem is an important topic.

Another important fact that should be mentioned is the case of an actual evidence of blood group change. This phenomenon is due to the transplantation. In real practice, isograft is hardly available. Therefore, the change of some blood antigen corresponding to the new engrafted marrow can be expected. Due to the recent advance on transplantation medicine and stem cell research the change of blood group is possible [70-71]. The blood group as a specific identification for an individual is therefore not a totally correct assumption.

REFERENCES

[1] Adachi T. Commemoration of Madam Curie. *Rinsho Hoshasen*. 1976 Jan;21(1):71-4.

[2] Dées de Sterio A. On the 100th birthday of Marie Curie (born November 7, 1867 in Warsaw). *Munch Med Wochenschr*. 1967 Nov 3;109(44):2332-3.

[3] Kyle RA, Shampo MA. Pierre Curie and Marie Curie-Sklodowska. *JAMA*. 1979 Jun 8;241(23):2511.

[4] Noble D. Marie Curie. Half-life of a legend. *Anal Chem*. 1993 Feb 15;65(4):215A-219A.

[5] Ial'tsev PD. Sixty-year anniversary of the discovery of roentgen rays. *Vestn Rentgenol Radiol*. 1956 Jan-Feb;31(1):3-7.

[6] Fedorova VA. Discovery of roentgen rays and their use in medicine. *Feldsher Akush*. 1955 Jul;(7):43-7.

[7] Berghoff E. History of the discovery of roentgen rays. *Wien Med Wochenschr*. 1956 Jan 21;106(3):71.

[8] Glocker R. Roentgen's discovery and its significance in medicine, science and technology. *Strahlentherapie*. 1952;87(1):1-6.

[9] Braendengen M, Tveit KM, Berglund A, Birkemeyer E, Frykholm G, Påhlman L, Wiig JN, Byström P, Bujko K, Glimelius B. Randomized phase III study comparing preoperative radiotherapy with chemoradiotherapy in nonresectable rectal cancer. *J Clin Oncol*. 2008 Aug 1;26(22):3687-94.

[10] Constantine C, Parhar P, Lymberis S, Fenton-Kerimian M, Han SC, Rosenstein BS, Formenti SC. Feasibility of accelerated whole-breast radiation in the treatment of patients with ductal carcinoma in situ of the breast. *Clin Breast Cancer.* 2008 Jun;8(3):269-74.

[11] Tsubokura M, Miura Y, Takei N, Kami M, Komatsu T. Radiotherapy hypofractionation in early breast cancer. *Lancet.* 2008 Jul 19;372(9634):204

[12] Ganswindt U, Stenzl A, Bamberg M, Belka C. Adjuvant radiotherapy for patients with locally advanced prostate cancer-a new standard? *Eur Urol.* 2008 Sep;54(3):528-42.

[13] Berk M. Radiation therapy as primary and adjuvant treatment for local and regional melanoma. *Cancer Control.* 2008 Jul;15(3):233-8.

[14] Sanfilippo NJ, Taneja SS, Chachoua A, Lepor H, Formenti SC. Phase I/II study of biweekly paclitaxel and radiation in androgen-ablated locally advanced prostate cancer. *J Clin Oncol.* 2008 Jun 20;26(18):2973-8.

[15] Mufazalov FF, Sakaeva DD, Shtefan AIu. Radiotherapy of malignant brain gliomas using teniposide. *Vopr Onkol.* 2008;54(2):208-10.

[16] Hughes S, Liong J, Miah A, Ahmad S, Leslie M, Harper P, Prendiville J, Shamash J, Subramaniam R, Gaya A, Spicer J, Landau D. A brief report on the safety study of induction chemotherapy followed by synchronous radiotherapy and cetuximab in stage III non-small cell lung cancer (NSCLC): SCRATCH study. *J Thorac Oncol.* 2008 Jun;3(6):648-51.

[17] Naito Y, Kubota K, Nihei K, Fujii T, Yoh K, Niho S, Goto K, Ohmatsu H, Saijo N, Nishiwaki Y. Concurrent chemoradiotherapy with cisplatin and vinorelbine for stage III non-small cell lung cancer. *J Thorac Oncol.* 2008 Jun;3(6):617-22.

[18] Ku GY, Ilson DH. Preoperative therapy in esophageal cancer. *Clin Adv Hematol Oncol.* 2008 May;6(5):371-9.

[19] Tsoutsou PG, Froudarakis ME, Bouros D, Koukourakis MI. Hypofractionated/accelerated radiotherapy with cytoprotection (HypoARC) combined with vinorelbine and liposomal doxorubicin for locally advanced non-small cell lung cancer (NSCLC). *Anticancer Res.* 2008 Mar-Apr;28(2B):1349-54.

[20] Barone C, Grillo R, Dongiovanni D, Birocco N, Rampino M, Redda MG, Garibaldi E, Munoz F, Pecorari G, Cavalot A, Garzinodemo P, Buffoni L, Ciuffreda L, Ricardi U, Cortesina G, Giordano C, Fasolis M, Berrone S, Bertetto O, Schena M. Induction chemotherapy followed by concurrent chemoradiotherapy in advanced head and neck squamous cell carcinoma. *Anticancer Res.* 2008 Mar-Apr;28(2B):1285-91.

[21] Yokoyama Y, Takano T, Nakahara K, Shoji T, Sato H, Yamada H, Yaegashi N, Okamura K, Kurachi H, Sugiyama T, Tanaka T, Sato A, Tase T, Mizunuma H. A phase II multicenter trial of concurrent chemoradiotherapy with weekly nedaplatin in advanced uterine cervical carcinoma: Tohoku Gynecologic Cancer Unit Study. *Oncol Rep.* 2008 Jun;19(6):1551-6.

[22] FitzGerald TJ, Urie M, Ulin K, Laurie F, Yorty J, Hanusik R, Kessel S, Jodoin MB, Osagie G, Cicchetti MG, Pieters R, McCarten K, Rosen N. Processes for quality improvements in radiation oncology clinical trials. *Int J Radiat Oncol Biol Phys.* 2008;71(1 Suppl):S76-9.

[23] Brizel DM, Murphy BA, Rosenthal DI, Pandya KJ, Glück S, Brizel HE, Meredith RF, Berger D, Chen MG, Mendenhall W. Phase II study of palifermin and concurrent chemoradiation in head and neck squamous cell carcinoma. *J Clin Oncol.* 2008 May 20;26(15):2489-96.

[24] Socinski MA, Blackstock AW, Bogart JA, Wang X, Munley M, Rosenman J, Gu L, Masters GA, Ungaro P, Sleeper A, Green M, Miller AA, Vokes EE. Randomized phase II trial of induction chemotherapy followed by concurrent chemotherapy and dose-escalated thoracic conformal radiotherapy (74 Gy) in stage III non-small-cell lung cancer: CALGB 30105. *J Clin Oncol.* 2008 May 20;26(15):2457-63.

[25] de Vreeze RS, de Jong D, Haas RL, Stewart F, van Coevorden F. Effectiveness of Radiotherapy in Myxoid Sarcomas is Associated with a Dense Vascular Pattern. *Int J Radiat Oncol Biol Phys.* 2008 Apr 28. [Epub ahead of print]

[26] Janaki MG, Nirmala S, Kadam AR, Ramesh BS, Sunitha KS. Epidural analgesia during brachytherapy for cervical cancer patients. *J Cancer Res Ther.* 2008 Apr-Jun;4(2):60-3.

[27] Papagelopoulos PJ, Mavrogenis AF, Mastorakos DP, Vlastou C, Vrouvas J, Soucacos PN. Free vascularised tissue transfer and brachytherapy for soft-tissue sarcomas of the extremities. *Injury.* 2008 Aug 5. [Epub ahead of print]

[28] Sedda AF, Rossi G, Cipriani C, Carrozzo AM, Donati P. Dermatological high-dose-rate brachytherapy for the treatment of basal and squamous cell carcinoma. *Clin Exp Dermatol.* 2008 Aug 2. [Epub ahead of print]

[29] Miura N, Kusuhara Y, Numata K, Shirato A, Hashine K, Sumiyoshi Y, Kataoka M, Takechi S. Radiation Pneumonitis Caused by a Migrated Brachytherapy Seed Lodged in the Lung. *Jpn J Clin Oncol.* 2008 Aug 2. [Epub ahead of print]

[30] Potter R, Kirisits C, Fidarova EF, Dimopoulos JC, Berger D, Tanderup K, Lindegaard JC. Present status and future of high-precision image guided adaptive brachytherapy for cervix carcinoma. *Acta Oncol.* 2008 Jul 25:1-12. [Epub ahead of print]

[31] Raisali G, Ghonchehnazi MG, Shokrani P, Sadeghi M. Monte Carlo and experimental characterization of the first AMIRS (103)Pd brachytherapy source. *Appl Radiat Isot.* 2008 Jun 14. [Epub ahead of print]

[32] Roessler B, Six LM, Gustorff B. Anaesthesia for brachytherapy. *Curr Opin Anaesthesiol.* 2008 Aug;21(4):514-8.

[33] Engle DB, Bradley KA, Chappell RJ, Conner JP, Hartenbach EM, Kushner DM. The Effect of Laparoscopic Guidance on Gynecologic Interstitial Brachytherapy. *J Minim Invasive Gynecol.* 2008 Jul 24. [Epub ahead of print]

[34] Mehdizadeh A, Fazelzadeh A, Karimi H. Alpha particle vascular brachytherapy in the treatment of in-stent Restenosis. *Int J Cardiol.* 2008 Jul 12. [Epub ahead of print]

[35] Semrau S, Kunz M, Baggesen K, Vogel H, Buchmann W, Gross G, Fietkau R. Successful treatment of field cancerization of the scalp by surface mould brachytherapy. *Br J Dermatol.* 2008 Jul 1. [Epub ahead of print

[36] Wojcik A, Buraczewska I, Sommer S, Brzozowska K, Pregowski J, Witkowski A, Garmol D, Pszona SA, Bulski W. Enhanced level of micronuclei in peripheral blood lymphocytes of patients treated for restenosis with (32)P endovascular brachytherapy. *Cardiovasc Revasc Med.* 2008 Jul-Sep;9(3):149-55.

[37] Fabrini MG, Perrone F, De Liguoro M, Cionini L. High-dose-rate brachytherapy in a large squamous cell carcinoma of the hand. *Brachytherapy*. 2008 Jul-Sep;7(3):270-5.

[38] Julow J, Kolumbán Z, Viola A, Major T, Kolumbán G. Prediction of volumetric change in the "triple ring" caused by glioma I-125 brachytherapy. *Neuro Oncol*. 2008 Aug;10(4):583-92.

[39] Ritter MA. Body mass index and prostate-specific antigen failure following brachytherapy for localized prostate cancer. *Urol Oncol*. 2008 Jul-Aug;26(4):448-9.

[40] Zhao YS, Yang HL, Liu CZ. Inhibitory effects of immunotargeting of Chinese cobra cytotoxin and iodine-131 against nasopharyngeal carcinoma cells in vitro. *Nan Fang Yi Ke Da Xue Xue Bao*. 2008 Jul;28(7):1235-6.

[41] Sanyal P, Bing-You RG, Braverman LE. Use of methotrexate to treat isolated Graves ophthalmopathy developing years after thyroidectomy and iodine 131 treatment of papillary thyroid cancer. *Endocr Pract*. 2008 May-Jun;14(4):422-5.

[42] Garsi JP, Schlumberger M, Rubino C, Ricard M, Labbé M, Ceccarelli C, Schvartz C, Henri-Amar M, Bardet S, de Vathaire F. Therapeutic administration of 131I for differentiated thyroid cancer: radiation dose to ovaries and outcome of pregnancies. *J Nucl Med*. 2008 May;49(5):845-52.

[43] Rajendran JG, Gopal AK, Fisher DR, Durack LD, Gooley TA, Press OW. Myeloablative 131I-tositumomab radioimmunotherapy in treating non-Hodgkin's lymphoma: comparison of dosimetry based on whole-body retention and dose to critical organ receiving the highest dose. *J Nucl Med*. 2008 May;49(5):837-44.

[44] Mäenpää HO, Heikkonen J, Vaalavirta L, Tenhunen M, Joensuu H. Low vs. high radioiodine activity to ablate the thyroid after thyroidectomy for cancer: a randomized study. *PLoS ONE*. 2008 Apr 2;3(4):e1885.

[45] Schaefer-Cutillo J, Friedberg JW. Non-myeloablative radioimmunotherapy for non-Hodgkin's lymphoma. *Semin Hematol*. 2008 Apr;45(2):110-7.

[46] Lau WY, Lai EC. Treatment of unresectable hepatocellular carcinoma with transarterial radioembolization: iodine-131-lipiodol. *ANZ J Surg*. 2008 May;78(5):331-2.

[47] Kim SJ, Choi HY, Kim IJ, Kim YK, Jun S, Nam HY, Kim JS. Limited cytoprotective effects of amifostine in high-dose radioactive iodine 131-treated well-differentiated thyroid cancer patients: analysis of quantitative salivary scan. *Thyroid*. 2008 Mar;18(3):325-31.

[48] de Kraker J, Hoefnagel KA, Verschuur AC, van Eck B, van Santen HM, Caron HN. Iodine-131-metaiodobenzylguanidine as initial induction therapy in stage 4 neuroblastoma patients over 1 year of age. *Eur J Cancer*. 2008 Mar;44(4):551-6.

[49] Nwosu AC, Jones L, Vora J, Poston GJ, Vinjamuri S, Pritchard DM. Assessment of the efficacy and toxicity of (131)I-metaiodobenzylguanidine therapy for metastatic neuroendocrine tumours. *Br J Cancer*. 2008 Mar 25;98(6):1053-8.

[50] Jerabek J, Dvorak M, Vojtisek B. Results of therapy of lower extremity ischemic disease by angiosurgery and radiointervention (PTA) methods. *Bratisl Lek Listy*. 2003;104(10):314-6.

[51] Black JH 3rd, LaMuraglia GM, Kwolek CJ, Brewster DC, Watkins MT, Cambria RP. Contemporary results of angioplasty-based infrainguinal percutaneous interventions. *J Vasc Surg*. 2005 Nov;42(5):932-9.

[52] Kuo WT, van den Bosch MA, Hofmann LV, Louie JD, Kothary N, Sze DY. Catheter-directed embolectomy, fragmentation, and thrombolysis for the treatment of massive pulmonary embolism after failure of systemic thrombolysis. *Chest*. 2008 Aug;134(2):250-4.

[53] Valpreda S, Messina M, Rabbia C. Stenting of transplant renal artery stenosis: outcome in a single center study. *J Cardiovasc Surg (Torino)*. 2008 Oct;49(5):565-70.

[54] Giller CA, Barnett DW, Thacker IC, Hise JH, Berger BD. Multidisciplinary treatment of a large cerebral dural arteriovenous fistula using embolization, surgery, and radiosurgery. *Proc (Bayl Univ Med Cent)*. 2008 Jul;21(3):255-7.

[55] Lee RW, Bakken AM, Palchik E, Saad WE, Davies MG. Long-term outcomes of endoluminal therapy for chronic atherosclerotic occlusive mesenteric disease. *Ann Vasc Surg*. 2008 Jul-Aug;22(4):541-6.

[56] Mansour M, Kamper L, Altenburg A, Haage P. Radiological central vein treatment in vascular access. *J Vasc Access*. 2008 Apr-Jun;9(2):85-101.

[57] Wang JB, Li MH, Fang C, Wang W, Cheng YS, Zhang PL, Du ZY, Wang J. Endovascular treatment of giant intracranial aneurysms with willis covered stents: technical case report. *Neurosurgery*. 2008 May;62(5):E1176-7.

[58] Gerszten PC, Burton SA, Ozhasoglu C, McCue KJ, Quinn AE. Radiosurgery for benign intradural spinal tumors. *Neurosurgery*. 2008 Apr;62(4):887-95

[59] Mathieu D, Kondziolka D, Flickinger JC, Fortin D, Kenny B, Michaud K, Mongia S, Niranjan A, Lunsford LD. Tumor bed radiosurgery after resection of cerebral metastases. *Neurosurgery*. 2008 Apr;62(4):817-23

[60] Fuller DB, Naitoh J, Lee C, Hardy S, Jin H. Virtual HDR CyberKnife treatment for localized prostatic carcinoma: dosimetry comparison with HDR brachytherapy and preliminary clinical observations. *Int J Radiat Oncol Biol Phys*. 2008 Apr 1;70(5):1588-97.

[61] Kondziolka D, Mathieu D, Lunsford LD, Martin JJ, Madhok R, Niranjan A, Flickinger JC. Radiosurgery as definitive management of intracranial meningiomas. *Neurosurgery*. 2008 Jan;62(1):53-8;

[62] Ryu S, Jin R, Jin JY, Chen Q, Rock J, Anderson J, Movsas B. Pain control by image-guided radiosurgery for solitary spinal metastasis. *J Pain Symptom Manage*. 2008 Mar;35(3):292-8.

[63] Franzin A, Vimercati A, Medone M, Serra C, Marzoli SB, Forti M, Gioia L, Valle M, Picozzi P. Neuroophthalmological evaluation after Gamma Knife surgery for cavernous sinus meningiomas. *Neurosurg Focus*. 2007;23(6):E10.

[64] Lekovic GP, Gonzalez LF, Shetter AG, Porter RW, Smith KA, Brachman D, Spetzler RF. Role of Gamma Knife surgery in the management of pineal region tumors. *Neurosurg Focus*. 2007;23(6):E12.

[65] Romanelli P, Wowra B, Muacevic A. Multisession CyberKnife radiosurgery for optic nerve sheath meningiomas. *Neurosurg Focus*. 2007;23(6):E11.

[66] Li G, Patil C, Adler JR, Lad SP, Soltys SG, Gibbs IC, Tupper L, Boakye M. CyberKnife rhizotomy for facetogenic back pain: a pilot study. *Neurosurg Focus.* 2007;23(6):E2.

[67] Pusztaszeri M, Villemure JG, Regli L, Do HP, Pica A. Radiosurgery for trigeminal neuralgia using a linear accelerator with BrainLab system: report on initial experience in Lausanne, Switzerland. *Swiss Med Wkly.* 2007 Dec 1;137(47-48):682-6.

[68] Taschner CA, Le Thuc V, Reyns N, Gieseke J, Gauvrit JY, Pruvo JP, Leclerc X. Gamma Knife surgery for arteriovenous malformations in the brain: integration of time-resolved contrast-enhanced magnetic resonance angiography into dosimetry planning. *Technical note. J Neurosurg.* 2007 Oct;107(4):854-9.

[69] Cho DY, Tsao M, Lee WY, Chang CS. Socioeconomic costs of open surgery and gamma knife radiosurgery for benign cranial base tumors. *Neurosurgery.* 2006 May;58(5):866-73.

[70] Koestner SC, Kappeler A, Schaffner T, Carrel TP, Nydegger UE, Mohacsi P. Histo-blood group type change of the graft from B to O after ABO mismatched heart transplantation. *Lancet.* 2004 May 8;363(9420):1523-5.

[71] Koestner SC, Kappeler A, Schaffner T, Carrel TP, Mohacsi PJ. ABO histo-blood group antigen expression on the graft endothelium long term after ABO-compatible, non-identical heart transplantation. *Xenotransplantation.* 2006 Mar;13(2):166-70.

Chapter VII

STEM CELL THERAPY

BEGINNING OF LIFE [1-3]

"God made the sun. God made the moon. God made the star." These sentences are basic principle for Christian. Living things in the worlds started for many million years ago. Nobody can tell the exact starting point of time for life. Life is complex. Generation of living thing is a very complicated process and no present high technology can work this. Natural makes life. This can be said that god made life. Due to Buddhism, life can be generated if there are fulfill criteria. as a) father and mother have sexual intercourse, b) the time is proper and c) there must be specific superstitious spirit for this condition. This is the fact. There must be gametes from both mother and father for fertilization. In human, beginning of new lie is widely studied. After fertilization, development process in utero is continuous. Embryonic generation is a developmental process for all human beings. Everyone in this world had to pass this step before birth. Further process as passing from embryo to fetus is the next step in utero. Birth is the finalized process for in utero processes and this is the starting point of human status.

Considering the embryonic period, the generation of cell and tissue is the main hallmark activity. Of several processes, first sign of life, movement, can be seen at the third month after fertilization. For cell and tissue growth, basic promoter as stem cell is required. Stem cell is the basic cell generator of other cells and tissues. This is also the important step in development for starting of complete life. Stem cell has its main function during in utero period. However, some stem cell is still existed and functional in full term human life. This can be seen in bone marrow, which is the source of generation of blood cell in circulation. It is accepted that blood cell must be generated all times thorough the life of human beings. Harvesting stem cell for medical use is the present focus. It can be important and applied for treatment process of some previously untreatable diseases. Stem cell technology could also be a significant helpful tool for an understanding on early human developmental process and screening potential candidates for new drug search.

Table 1. Summary on important steps of development in embryology

Period	Details
Fertilization (day 0)	This is the process that male gamete or spermatozoa penetrate into egg or female gamete to internally fertilize. The fertilized egg will be moved to implant into the internal wall of uterus.
9th week after fertilization	Some organ formations can be seen.
11th week after fertilization	Shoulder can be visualized. Rib and spine formation from cartilage can be observed.
12th week after fertilization	The first sign of life, moving, can be seen. After this stage, embryo will be called fetus.

BASIC CONCEPTS OF STEM CELL THERAPY

Stem cell therapy is a new concept in medical science. This treatment concept is the use of cell for cell therapy. Application of progenitor to specific defective part aiming at the regenerative for treatment of specific pathological condition is the main concept of stem cell therapy. This approach is a novel treatment and under trialed. Indeed, stem cell is known for years. However, the introduction of stem cell therapy for treatment in medicine is a new thing. Historically, classical approach to derive new human embryonic stem cell line includes the harvest of the inner cell mass from a human embryo. However, this cannot avoid destroying the embryo and raise the critical ethical issue. As previously mentioned, the first sign of first begins at 12th week after fertilization and this is called embryo status [4-5]. There should be a necessity to re-address the issue of when life begins and the dignity of human embryos [4-5].

The other approach to derive a new human embryonic stem cell line is from somatic cell nuclear transfer (SCNT) technique or cloning technique. This famous technique is firstly used previously in reported on magic cloned Dolly sheep. This method was accepted be a good potential candidate for providing patient-specific stem cell line that would be used for transplantation without possible problem on rejection due to immune system [4-5]. Presenting, this approach has not been proved successful in human for many reasons. The main ethical concern is that cloning brings several ethical problems. Who will be the mother and father? Religiously, this is also cross the acceptable principle. Cloning human for harvest organ to treat the other is totally unacceptable. In addition to the somatic cell nuclear transfer or cloning technique, a new mean that based on using donor nucleus for nuclear transfer has been modified to prevent the implantation potential of the embryo created and this can manage the ethical problem [4-5]. This is a present acceptable modification. This is also the basement for concept of present stem cell therapy.

Briefly, the concept for each stem cell therapy can be as the followings:

a) Harvesting of Stem Cell

Harvesting of stem cell is the first step for collection of stem cell for further medical usage. In adult, as previously mentioned, the most important source of stem cell is the borne marrow because stem cell is stem cell is still existed in bone marrow for generation of blood cell in blood circulation. Therefore, the basic medical procedure for stem cell collection in adult is bone marrow aspiration. This should be performed by well trained clinical pathologist or hematologist. The site for bone marrow collection is iliac crest. Presently, there is another new way for collection of stem cell. This makes use of cord blood and called cord blood stem cell collection. This can be done without invasive procedure to the donor. This is mainly used in many setting. More details on cord blood collection will be further described in this chapter.

b) Storage of Stem Cell

Storage of stem cell is usually required because stem cell is usually not suddenly used after stem cell collection. Therefore, there must be a process to prepare and store stem cell for future usage. Before storage, stem cell must be typed by typing technique for all basic parameters. It must also be cleaned. At present, there many commercial stem cell storage center and stem cell bank.

c) Usage of Stem Cell

Usage of stem cell is the final step. When it is indicated and there is no contraindication for stem cell therapy, stem cell should be ordered from the bank for usage. For using stem cell it must be well matched and prepared. Basically, it must be conditioned and promoted for further development into target desired cells specific for each treatment. This steps makes used of many advanced biotechnology procedures. The success of any stem cell treatment is usually determined by this step.

As a conclusion, stem cell therapy has been accepted as an emerging technology that could change the present approach toward curing many chronic disorders and degenerative conditions. As previously mentioned, stem cell therapy can be applied for regenerative medicine which is another promising area of medical therapy for the coming years. Cell and tissue replacement therapy could be the final solution for present several incurable diseases. However, stem cell therapy also brings up many controversial issues from the medical ethics. This will be further discussed in this article.

For example, there are many arguments on the

Medical Ethics for Stem Cell Therapy

Because stem cell is a new technology it is a focused area in medical ethics.

It should be noted that justification to destroy one life, either an human embryo, to save another life or candidate for stem cell therapy is a big question. This is a good ethical dilemma scenario of the situation when science intersects with standard ethical principles.

The appropriate solution must be a mid way position that would support the advancement of science for the benefit of human, while maintaining the ethics. This balance status would be a key success for sustainable science and society development for real application of stem cell technology. Kiatpongsan and Pruksananonda said that there were common concerns for bioethics in stem cell technology as a). There must be a respect for human dignity, b) There must be a respect for life that implied limiting growth of blastocyst to 12 weeks when a primitive streak was formed, c) There must be an autonomy or informed consent from embryo donors, d) There must be a donor and recipient privacy and confidentiality, e) There must be a non-commercializatio, f) There must be a limitation to research for therapeutic purposes, g) There must be an ethics review before commencement of the research and h) There must be a traceability of cell lines used in both research and clinical practice for safety and quality assurance [6]. Some important reports on medical ethics for stem cell therapy will be listed in Table 2.

Table 2. Some important reports on medical ethics for stem cell therapy

authors	details
Baylis and McLeod [7]	Baylis and McLeod put a debate on the buying and selling of eggs for stem cell research [7]. Baylis and McLeod said that the focused debate was on the topic tha women should be paid a fair wage for their reproductive labor or tissues, while others argue against the further commodification of reproductive labor and worry about voluntariness among potential egg donors [7].
Daley et al. [8]	Daley et al. proposed a guideline for human embryonic stem cell research [8].
Sadeghi [9]	Sadeghi proposed on islamic perspectives on human cloning [9]. Sadeghi said that human cloning for biomedical research and exploitation of stem cells from cloned embryos at the blastocyst stage for therapeutic purposes might be acceptable [9].
Outomuro [10]	Outomuro discussed on moral dilemmas around a global human embryonic stem cell bank [10].
Ecker and O'Rourke [11]	Ecker and O'Rourke noted that banking embryonic stem cells for solid organ transplantation was problematic and premature [11].
Ross and Philipson [12]	Ross and Philipson discussed on ethics of hematopoietic stem cell transplantation in type 1 diabetes mellitus [12].
Silani and Cova [13]	Silani and Cova discussed on ethics of stem cell therapy in multiple sclerosis [13].
Bongaerts and Severijnen [14]	Bongaerts and Severijnen discussed on oocyte donation for stem cell research [14].

Cord Blood Stem Cell Collection

A. General Introduction

After birth, once the child's umbilical cord is clamped, a small volume of residual blood remains in the umbilical cord [15]. This can be collected into a special blood bag and then taken for further storage and processing [15]. As the collection of the umbilical cord blood was performed after the baby's birth, it does not affect the baby's birth and also no harm is caused to the baby or the mother [15-21]. An acceptable usage of cord blood is as an alternative to bone marrow as a source of hematopoietic stem cells for allogeneic transplantation to siblings or to unrelated recipients [22-23]. Any women can donate cord blood for unrelated recipients to public cord blood banks [22-23]. However, the emerging medical ethics problem in cord blood collection is the issue of commercial cord blood banking as previously mentioned [24-25]. According to the Working Group on Ethical Issues in Umbilical Cord Blood Banking, umbilical cord blood banking for autologous use related to greater uncertainty than banking for allogeneic use, marketing practices for umbilical cord blood banking in the private sector need close attention and the process of obtaining informed consent for collection of umbilical cord blood had to be completed before labor and delivery [25]. Allogeneic cord blood transplantations is used in the hematology and oncology area [26]. Cord blood banks, either public or from non-profit corporations, can be seen in several countries Umbilical cord blood can be collected and stored frozen for many years [22].

B. Cord Blood Collection Procedure

Cord blood collection should be performed within a total quality system and good manufacturing practice facilities. Protocols should be set based upon risk assessment and cost efficiency [27]. It is recommended that cord blood collection needed to be after the permission for cord blood donation [28]. Surbek et al. reported a high acceptance of umbilical cord blood donation for banking and stem cell transplantation purposes in pregnant women without previous knowledge background [29]. As there are no major discrepancies between women of different ethnic background, a high degree of diversity of HLA-types of donated cord blood samples can be expected and may lead to the underrepresentation of ethnic minorities in bone marrow donor records [29]. Danzer et al. reported a high degree of satisfaction of unrelated umbilical cord blood donation for banking in women half a year after delivery [30]. Despite a well-performed and detailed informed consent procedure, one of the ongoing considerable aspects for the donators in cord blood banking are the concern regarding of improper use of the cells, such as genetic laboratory testing [30]. Accurate and detailed counseling of pregnant women and their partners therefore can increase the likelihood that they will donate cord blood for unrelated banking.

For cord blood collection, there are at least 3 means: Method 1 = Hanging method after delivering the placenta, Method 2 = Aspiration from in utero placenta, Method 3 = Aspiration from in utero placenta and Syringe-assisted aspiration. Wacharaprechanont et al. recently performed a comparative study on the 3 methods using the closed system and showed that final one was the best method but it required more trained personnel and involved a complicated procedure [31]. After collection, the quality of the cord blood (volume, total white blood cells (WBC) count, CD34+ and sterility control) needed to be checked. According to a recent study from Thailand, the quality of the cord blood collected by any methods was satisfactory and discard rate of collecting units were comparable with those reported from other cord blood banks [31]. However, Wong et al. found that the reduction of stem and progenitor cells correlated significantly with that of major cell populations, indicating a general cell loss, possibly owing to clotting activities developed with time [32]. They documented strong evidence for recommending the collection of cord blood before the placental birth [33]. At present, the ex utero collection is more widely used. Basically, the umbilical vein is punctured or catheterized, and then cord blood must be aspirated with syringes contained anticoagulants [34]. Another method is to drain blood into a collection-bag by gravity [34]. The collection bags with anticoagulants provided by TERUMO and BAXTER HEALTHCARE CO [34]. Askari et al. said that donor selection and collection technique modifications might increase product quality [35]. They noted that total nucleated cell count was more affected by different variables than CD34+ count [35].

Table 3. Basic methods for cord blood collection

Methods	Details
1. Hanging method after placental birth	The umbilical cord blood is collected after the placental birth [36]. The entire collection process takes places after the umbilical cord is clamped off from the newborn [36]. The placenta is then placed into a sterile device with the umbilical cord hanging through [36]. The cord blood is collected by draining the cord blood with the help of gravity [36]. In this case, they can usually collect between 40 and 150 milliliters of blood [36]
2. Direct aspiration from in utero placenta	The cord blood is got from the umbilical vein with 20-mL syringes while the placenta still attaches in utero [36].
3. Direct aspiration from in utero placenta and syringe-assisted aspiration	The collection of cord blood involved direct aspiration by direct puncture of the ethanol-sterilized umbilical vein at a site distal to the placenta, to decrease to a minimum the feasibility of cross-contamination by lymphocytes from mother [36].

C. Cord Blood Banking

To establish a cord blood bank, a big panel of frozen, HLA-typed cord blood units storage is required. Cryopreserved, unprocessed cord blood units need vast storage space. Various techniques can be used to isolate stem and progenitor cells from cord blood to reduce the volume of blood. The described methods include hydroxyethyl starch sedimentation (HES) with two centrifugation steps, and the top and bottom (T&B) isolation of buffy coat following a single centrifugation, and filter systems for processing cord blood. The hydroxyethyl starch method and the T & B method can be for the volume reduction of human placental and umbilical cord blood units [36]. The new filter system was proved to be efficient for placenta cord blood processing, encompassing a very simple handling procedure with a favorable recovery of haematopoietic progenitor cells [36]. Takahashi et al. indicated that filters that capture stem and progenitor cells might be a proper methodology for processing cord blood collected for banking [37]. Dal Cortivo et al. proposed that Procord was a good method for erythrocyte depletion of cord blood, and recoveries of nucleated cells and progenitor cells were comparable to those cells derived from similar processing [37]. Nevertheless, as all existing methods, it is related to cell and progenitor cell loss [38]. At present, automated system for reduction of blood volume is also available. Armitage et al. studied using the Optipress II Automated Blood Component Extractor (Opti II) from Baxter Healthcare Corporation, to decrease the volume of the cord blood collection, preserving the quantity and quality of the progenitor cells, in a closed system [39]. They reported that using this technique for processing cord blood units decreased storage requirement by two-thirds but preserves the quantity and quality of the progenitor cells [39]. Solves et al. recently compared two different means for CB volume reduction in both development and routine phases: HES sedimentation and T & B fractionation with the Optipress II [40]. According to this work, the volume reduction method with the Optipress II was a time-saving system that permitted good cell recoveries [40]. In contrast, the main advantage of the HES method is the higher RBC depletion that affects CFU content [40]. Reducing RBC content should be the main aim of further improvements for volume reduction using the Optipress II method [40].

Although placental blood has recently been a new available source of hematopoietic progenitors for marrow replacement, limited attention has been provided to systems suitable to ensure the short-term and long-term quality of placental blood units applied for transplantation [41]. For cord blood banking, quality system is needed [41-42]. It includes the organizational structure, procedures, processes and resources required to implement quality management [41-42]. The number of cord blood banks throughout the world is increasing rapidly [41-42]. In the USA and Europe, more than ten thousands placental cord blood units are stored and available for possible transplantation at present [41-42]. The practices of umbilical cord blood collection, mother selection, infectious disease screening, cell manipulation and storage needs to be standardized [43]. Some accreditation process should be set as an important key for assessing operating procedures and the quality assurance programs of the banks, and for allowing the international exchange of placental blood between transplant centers. Several medical ISOs can be applied [41-42]. The Quality System must be used and subjected to external audit at regular intervals so that certification is guaranteed [41-42].

Transcription Factor Binding Site E2F Transcription Factor: A Prediction

As previously mentioned, there are complex processes in generation of adult cells from stem cell. Transcriptional factor is a focus. However, the knowledge on this area is limited. The application of bioinformatics can be helpful in this step. Here, an example will be hereby presented. E2F transcription factoris an important regulator of genes needed for appropriate progression through the cell cycle, and in special situations [43]. E2F associated co-activators promote activating histone marks whereas recruitment of co-repressors associated with E2F brings accretion of inhibitory histone modifications that provoke chromatin compaction [44]. It can be said that E2Fs help initiate both cell proliferation and cell death [43]. It has been reported that cell cycle assist of stem cells is controlled through inhibition of E2F activity [45]. The study on the expression of E2F is important in stem cell medicine at present. Basically, E2F contributes to the transcriptional activation of many genes as previously described. Study of transcription factor binding site within E2Fcan valuably complement experimental detection. In this work, the author determined transcription factor binding site in E2F transcription factor. This work aims to characterize transcription factor binding sites in the sequence of the transcription factor E2F. This approach is interesting and may well contribute to our understanding of how E2F transcription is regulated.

```
GATCTTACAATTGATTTGAATATGGCTGTCAACGATTTAGGAGTTCAGAAG
AGAAGAATATACGATATAACAAATGTATTAGAAGGAATAGGTTACATTGA
AAAAATCTCAAAAAACAAA  120

ATTAAATGGGTAGGTGCCACTGATAATCCATAACTGGAAACAGAGCTCTA
ATAGATTAAATAAGAATTGGAATAACTGTAAAATGAAGAAAAAACATAC
GATTTTTGGATTGAGCACTTA  240

TAAAAAAATCTATAAGACAAGTTTCAGACCGAACCTGAAATCGCTAAATA
CACATTTCTAACCTAAGAGGACTTTAAGGAGCTCTCCAAAAGTTAGTAAA
TTGATCATAAAGGTGAAACT  360

TTATTTATTATTACTGCTCCTAAAGGCACATTAGTAGAAACCGTATTGGAA
AATAATCCTGAATATCCTTATTAAGTCTACTTAAATAGCTCGAAAGTGCAG
GGTTAAAATAATGAAATT  480
1          ------------>V$OCT1_Q6(0.92)
2                      ------------>V$EVI1_04(0.86)

CAAGTCTTCATTTGTTAAGATGAAAATTATCCAATCGAATATGATAGGAA
ATAGAAATGACATAATTAATTCAATTATTATAAAATTTTGCAGCATTCCAT
AAAACCTTAAATGATTTAC  600
AACATTTTTGATCA
```

Figure 1. Predicted transciption factor binding site in E2F transcription factor.

The prediction of transcription factor binding site in E2F transcription factor was performed using in silico transcription factor binding site analysis.The tool for matrix search for transcription factor binding sitesnamely MATCH was used. According to this work, the input is the sequence of E2F.Briefly, MATCH [46] is designed for searching transcription factor binding sites in DNA sequences using baseline database, TRANSFAC [47]. The MATCH algorithm uses two parameters to score putative matches to the baseline database: the matrix similarity score and the core similarity score [47].These scores imply the binding affinities within molecules [47]. The cut off levels of the two parameters in this work are 0.7 and 0.75, respectively. These levels were set in order to minimize false positive. Identified transcription factors will match to their high-affinity binding sites. The output is the detected transcription factor binding sites. In addition, the frequency of sites per nucleotide (basepair) is also calculated. According to this study, there are two detected transcription factor binding sites (Figure 1). The frequency of sites per nucleotide is equal to 0.003257(2 sites per 614 basepairs).The first identified site is V$OCT1_Q6 (496taagatGAAAAttat510, core value = 0.893, matrix value = 0.916). The second identified site is V$EVI1_04(517gaatatgatAGGAAa531,core value = 0.776, matrix value = 0.861).

The role of E2F in the mammalian cell cycle is confirmed [48].Cell cycle-dependent transcriptional repression of the E2F promoters is controlled through E2F-binding sites and nearby corepressor site [49].Tavner et al. reported that targeting an E2F site in the mouse genome inhibits promoter silencing in quiescent and post-mitotic cells [50].In addition, Rayman et al. reported that E2F mediated cell cycle-dependent transcriptional repression in vivo by recruitment of an HDAC1/mSin3B corepressor complex [51].Here, the author tried to determine the transciption factor binding sites within E2F. Two sites, Oct-1 and Evi-1, are determined.Oct-1 is a member of the POU protein family helping in the activation of snRNA promoters and some mRNA promoters [52]. Oct-1 also cooperatively transactivates PU.1 designing cell fate between mast cells and monocytes [52]. Evi-1 is a transcription factor with two sets ozinc finger domains [53]. The temporally and spatially restricted pattern of Evi-1 expression in embryonic tissues implies a significant role of Evi-1 in organogenesis and morphogenesis in development [54-55]. The two identified binding sites to Oct-1 and Evi-1 that E2F is important in stem cell development in normal and pathological process.

REFERENCES

[1] Fetal growth and maternal nutrition. *Nutr Rev.* 1972 Oct;30(10):226-9.

[2] Nalbandov AV, Cook B. Reproduction. *Annu Rev Physiol.* 1968;30:245-78.

[3] Agostoni E. Preimplantation development of the mammalian embryo. *Ann Ist Super Sanita.* 1993;29(1):15-25.

[4] Kiatpongsan S, Tannirandon Y, Numchaisrikha P, Rungsiwiwat R. Conventional and novel methods for embryonic stem cell line derivation. *J Med Assoc Thai* 2006; 89: 896-903.

[5] Green RM. Can we develop ethically universal embryonic stem-cell lines? *Nat Rev Genet* 2007; 8: 480-5.

[6] Kiatpongsan S, Pruksananonda K. International trends in bioethics for embryonic stem cell research. *J Med Assoc Thai.* 2006 Sep;89(9):1542-4.

[7] Baylis F, McLeod C. The stem cell debate continues: the buying and selling of eggs for research. *J Med Ethics.* 2007 Dec;33(12):726-31.

[8] Daley GQ, Ahrlund Richter L, Auerbach JM, Benvenisty N, Charo RA, Chen G, Deng HK, Goldstein LS, Hudson KL, Hyun I, Junn SC, Love J, Lee EH, McLaren A, Mummery CL, Nakatsuji N, Racowsky C, Rooke H, Rossant J, Schöler HR, Solbakk JH, Taylor P, Trounson AO, Weissman IL, Wilmut I, Yu J, Zoloth L. Ethics. The ISSCR guidelines for human embryonic stem cell research. *Science.* 2007 Feb 2;315(5812):603-4.

[9] Sadeghi M. Islamic perspectives on human cloning. *Hum Reprod Genet Ethics.* 2007;13(2):32-40.

[10] Outomuro D. Moral dilemmas around a global human embryonic stem cell bank. *Am J Bioeth*. 2007 Aug;7(8):47-8

[11] Ecker JL, O'Rourke PP. An immodest proposal: banking embryonic stem cells for solid organ transplantation is problematic and premature. *Am J Bioeth*. 2007 Aug;7(8):48-50

[12] Ross LF, Philipson LH. Ethics of hematopoietic stem cell transplantation in type 1 diabetes mellitus. *JAMA*. 2007 Jul 18;298(3):285.

[13] Silani V, Cova L. Stem cell transplantation in multiple sclerosis: safety and ethics. *J Neurol Sci*. 2008 Feb 15;265(1-2):116-21.

[14] Bongaerts GP, Severijnen RS. Oocyte donation for stem cell research. *Science*. 2007 Apr 20;316(5823):368-70.

[15] What is Cord Blood? Available online at www.cordbloodbankingguide.com

[16] Mott JC. Control of the foetal circulation. *J Exp Biol*. 1982 Oct;100:129-46.

[17] Edelstone DI. Regulation of blood flow through the ductus venosus. *J Dev Physiol*. 1980 Aug;2(4):219-38.

[18] Kunzel W. Umbilical circulation--physiology and pathology. *J Perinat Med*. 1981;9 Suppl 1:68-71.

[19] Mayani H, Alvarado-Moreno JA, Flores-Guzman P. Biology of human hematopoietic stem and progenitor cells present in circulation. *Arch Med Res*. 2003 Nov-Dec;34(6):476-88.

[20] Elhassani SB. The umbilical cord: care, anomalies, and diseases. *South Med J*. 1984 Jun;77(6):730-6.

[21] Fyle J. Routine commercial umbilical cord blood collection. *RCM Midwives*. 2006 Jul;9(7):261.

[22] Fisk NM, Roberts IA, Markwald R, Mironov V. Can routine commercial cord blood banking be scientifically and ethically justified? *PLoS Med*. 2005 Feb;2(2):e44.

[23] Drew D. Umbilical cord blood banking. *Adv Nurse Pract*. 2005 Apr;13(4):Suppl 2-6.

[24] Kusminsky G. Umbilical cord blood criopreservation for autologous use. An ethical problem. *Medicina (B Aires)*. 2006;66(4):367-71.

[25] Sugarman J, Kaalund V, Kodish E, Marshall MF, Reisner EG, Wilfond BS, Wolpe PR. Ethical issues in umbilical cord blood banking. Working Group on Ethical Issues in Umbilical Cord Blood Banking. *JAMA*. 1997 Sep 17;278(11):938-43.

[26] Dalle JH. Cord blood banking: public versus private banks--facts to ponder and consider. *Arch Pediatr*. 2005 Mar;12(3):298-304.

[27] Warwick RM, Barbara JA. Safety aspects of cord blood banking. *Bone Marrow Transplant*. 1998 Jun;21 Suppl 3:S40-2.

[28] Kommission Qualitatssicherung der Schweizerischen Gesellschaft fur Gynakologie und Geburtshilfe. Umbilical cord blood donation: unrelated donation, familial (directed) donation and autologous donation (private banking) *Gynakol Geburtshilfliche Rundsch*. 2003 Apr;43(2):118-21.

[29] Surbek DV, Islebe A, Schonfeld B, Tichelli A, Gratwohl A, Holzgreve W. Umbilical cord blood transplantation: acceptance of umbilical cord blood donation by pregnant patients. *Schweiz Med Wochenschr*. 1998 May 2;128(18):689-95

[30] Danzer E, Holzgreve W, Troeger C, Kostka U, Steimann S, Bitzer J, Gratwohl A, Tichelli A, Seelmann K, Surbek DV. Attitudes of Swiss mothers toward unrelated umbilical cord blood banking 6 months after donation. *Transfusion.* 2003 May;43(5):604-8.

[31] Wacharaprechanont T, O-Charoen R, Vanichsetakul P, Sudjai D, Kupatawintu P, Seksarn P, Samritpradit P, Charoenvidhya D. Cord blood collection for the National Cord Blood Bank in Thailand. *J Med Assoc Thai.* 2003 Jun;86 Suppl 2:S409-16.

[32] Cord blood collection. Available online at http://www.cordplan.com/en/cord-blood-collection.html

[33] Wong A, Yuen PM, Li K, Yu AL, Tsoi WC. Cord blood collection before and after placental delivery: levels of nucleated cells, haematopoietic progenitor cells, leukocyte subpopulations and macroscopic clots. *Bone Marrow Transplant.* 2001 Jan;27(2):133-8.

[34] Ohnuma K, Nishihira H. Harvest techniques for cord blood after delivery of placenta. *Rinsho Byori.* 1999 May;Suppl 110:21-7.

[35] Askari S, Miller J, Chrysler G, McCullough J. Impact of donor- and collection-related variables on product quality in ex utero cord blood banking. *Transfusion.* 2005 Feb;45(2):189-94.

[36] Yasutake M, Sumita M, Terashima S, Tokushima Y, Nitadori Y, Takahashi TA. Stem cell collection filter system for human placental/umbilical cord blood processing. *Vox Sang.* 2001 Feb;80(2):101

[37] Takahashi TA, Rebulla P, Armitage S, van Beckhoven J, Eichler H, Kekomaki R, Letowska M, Wahab F, Moroff G. Multi-laboratory evaluation of procedures for reducing the volume of cord blood: influence on cell recoveries. *Cytotherapy.* 2006;8(3):254-64.

[38] Dal Cortivo L, Robert I, Mangin C, Sameshima T, Kora S, Gluckman E, Benbunan M, Marolleau JP. Cord blood banking: volume reduction using "Procord" Terumo filter. *J Hematother Stem Cell Res.* 2000 Dec;9(6):885-90.

[39] Armitage S, Fehily D, Dickinson A, Chapman C, Navarrete C, Contreras M. Cord blood banking: volume reduction of cord blood units using a semi-automated closed system. *Bone Marrow Transplant.* 1999 Mar;23(5):505-9.

[40] Solves P, Mirabet V, Planelles D, Blasco I, Perales A, Carbonell-Uberos F, Soler MA, Roig R. Red blood cell depletion with a semiautomated system or hydroxyethyl starch sedimentation for routine cord blood banking: a comparative study. *Transfusion.* 2005 Jun;45(6):867-73.

[41] Sirchia G, Rebulla P, Lecchi L, Mozzi F, Crepaldi R, Parravicini A. Implementation of a quality system (ISO 9000 series) for placental blood banking. *J Hematother.* 1998 Feb;7(1):19-35.

[42] Sirchia G, Rebulla P, Mozzi F, Lecchi L, Lazzari L, Ratti I. A quality system for placental blood banking. *Bone Marrow Transplant.* 1998 Jun;21 Suppl 3:S43-7.

[43] Iaquinta PJ, Lees JA. Life and death decisions by the E2F transcription factors. *Curr Opin Cell Biol.* 2007 Dec;19(6):649-57.

[44] Blais A, Dynlacht BD. E2F-associated chromatin modifiers and cell cycle control. *Curr Opin Cell Biol.* 2007 Dec;19(6):658-62.

[45] Furukawa Y. Cell cycle regulation of hematopoietic stem cells. *Hum Cell.* 1998 Jun;11(2):81-92.

[46] Kel AE, G?ssling E, Reuter I, Cheremushkin E, Kel-Margoulis OV, Wingender E. MATCH: A tool for searching transcription factor binding sites in DNA sequences. *Nucleic Acids Res.* 2003 Jul 1;31(13):3576-9.

[47] Matys V, Fricke E, Geffers R, G?ssling E, Haubrock M, Hehl R, Hornischer K, Karas D, Kel AE, Kel-Margoulis OV, Kloos DU, Land S, Lewicki-Potapov B, Michael H, M?nch R, Reuter I, Rotert S, Saxel H, Scheer M, Thiele S, Wingender E. TRANSFAC: transcriptional regulation, from patterns to profiles. *Nucleic Acids Res.* 2003 Jan 1;31(1):374-8.

[48] Moran E. The role of E2F in the mammalian cell cycle. *Biochim Biophys Acta.* 1993 Aug 23;1155(2):125-31.

[49] Nakajima Y, Yamada S, Kamata N, Ikeda MA.Interaction of E2F-Rb family members with corepressors binding to the adjacent E2F site. *Biochem Biophys Res Commun.* 2007 Dec 28;364(4):1050-5.

[50] Tavner F, Frampton J, Watson RJ. Targeting an E2F site in the mouse genome prevents promoter silencing in quiescent and post-mitotic cells. *Oncogene.* 2007 Apr 26;26(19):2727-35.

[51] Rayman JB, Takahashi Y, Indjeian VB, Dannenberg JH, Catchpole S, Watson RJ, te Riele H, Dynlacht BD.E2F mediates cell cycle-dependent transcriptional repression in vivo by recruitment of an HDAC1/mSin3B corepressor complex. *Genes Dev.* 2002 Apr 15;16(8):933-47.

[52] Pankratova EV, Deyev IE, Zhenilo SV, Polanovsky OL.Tissue-specific. *Mol Genet Genomics.* isoforms of the ubiquitous transcription factor Oct-1. 2001 Oct;266(2):239-45.

[53] Nishiyama C. Molecular mechanism of allergy-related gene regulation and hematopoietic cell development by transcription factors. *Biosci Biotechnol Biochem.* 2006 Jan;70(1):1-9.

[54] Hirai H.The transcription factor Evi-1. *Int J Biochem Cell Biol.* 1999 Dec;31(12):1367-71.

[55] The EVI-1 gene--its role in pathogenesis of human leukemias. *Leuk Res.* 2000 Jul;24(7):553-8.

Chapter VIII

ADVENT IN TRANSFUSION MEDICINE

INTRODUCTION TO BLOOD COMPONENT IN MEDICINE [1]

A. Introduction

There are many basic case groups to receive extensive blood transfusions including the cases in intensive care unit, thalassemic cases, acute blood lost cases as well as traumatic cases. Approximately four-fifth get multiple transfusions. At present donor exposure is an issue because transfusion risk is still apparent [2]. Gived blood should be applied for the treatment of cases as well as poses well asled with the same serious respect as well as ethical stas well asards as with which it was gived by the donor. Directed donor or purcposesed system should not be encouraged. Anonymous donation should be applied. As a rule blood msut be given as a gift with no reimbursement as well as should be applied to an unknown case with the intention to help as well as not to harm [2]. Donation shall be easy as well as secure for the donor. Therefore, blood shall be poses well asled with respect as well as should be applied with the intension to treat cases as previouly stated. Promotion of the blood donation is the topic. Owing to a recent study, the principal obstacle for blood donation is fear owing to poor knowledge [3].

Gived blood have to be applied for treatment of case directly or indirectly. Direct help to the case might be transfusion of single units or transfusion of units from a batch, platelets or plasma outcomes. Indirect help to the case include using of a few tubes for laboratory controls or many units for stas well asards with the intention to help cases to set normal values for a new test which is useful for laboratory medicine. Use of gived blood for other aims than transfusion have to be no specific information when blood is applied as laboratory quality controls but information for other kinds of use as well as assure for no identification at the pposese of informed consent with identification of donor is needed [2].

B. Risk of Transfusions

Acute hemolytic (immediate antibody-antigen reactive action triggered by transfusion of ABO incompatible blood) as well as delayed hemolytic (sensitization to minor blood group antigens during a previous transfusion which results in a reactive action 3 to 10 days after a subsequent transfusion) are the two most common complicated outcomes of blood transfusion [4]. The third kind is febrile, non-hemolytic owing to reactive action between antibodies as well as LEUKOCYTE antigens or plasma proteins [5]. It should be noted that all three kinds are rare in the newborn because of a defect in isohemagglutins as well as poor antibody response to alien antigens. In addition, blood transfusion also had the risk for transmission of many blood borne pathogenic agents [6] including syphilis, HIV 1, HIV 2, Human T-lymphotrophic virus 1 (HTLV-1), hepatitis B surface antigen (HbsAg),malaria, microfilaria as well as babesia. These pathogenic agents should be screened in the basic blood transfusion screening test. Also, some new biomarkers are introduced including hepatitis C virus (HCV), alanine aminotransferase (ALT), a surrogate biomarker for HIV infection, as well as hepatitis B core antibody (Anti HBc), a surrogate biomarker for non-A, non-B hepatitis. According to the stas well asard of Thai National Blood Bank, the donor screening tests include ABO grouping, Rh, HBsAg, Anti HIV, Anti HCV, VDRL as well as malaria.

The rare complicated outcomes include graft versus host disease (GVHD) [7-8] which usually occurs 4 to 30 days after a transfusion as well as associated with high fatality. Concerning the pathophysiology, T-lymphocytes in a transfusion product engraft in the recipient as well as react to the recipients tissues. The clinical pictures included liver dysfunction, watery diarrhea, erythroderma as well as pancytopenia. This condition is firstly described in immunocompromised children as well as noticed most recently in cases who received blood gived by relatives. The new suggestion for prevention of graft versus host disease is irradiation [9-10]. The irradiation is indicated in knownsuspected immunodefect case getting blood from biologic relative as section of a directed donor program. It is also indicated in in utero or exchange transfusion, bone marrow transplant recipients, infants with malignancies (leukemia, neuroblastomas), very not high birth weight infants, infants getting blood components with large amounts of leukocytes (platelets, granulocyte transfusions), cases with absolute lymphopenia (lymphocytes < 500). It should be noted that removal of lymphocytes by white blood cell (LEUKOCYTE) filter is not a replacement for irradiation. Irradiated red blood cell can be stored for 28 days or equal to the age of the principal irradiated blood components based on which date is earlier. Irradiate blood should be washed prior to administration to remove excessive potassium leaking out of the red blood cell. However, it should be mentioned that both irradiation as well as leukocyte filtering are not the method to prevent all transfusion reactive actions since there are other causes of transfusion reactive actions.

C. Indications for Transfusions

There are many indications [11] including replacing phlebotomy losses, treatment of symptomatic cardiac disease, treatment of severe respiratory distressed syndrome, surgical management, replacement of acute blood loss as well as exchange transfusion (in some diseases such as malaria as well as leptospirosis). Concerning the administration issues, cardiovascular system can only poses well asle acute maximizes of 10 to 15% without compromise. Most units use single transfusion volumes of 10 to 20% over 2 to 6 hours as well as dose of blood applied is determined by hematocrit of donor blood. Freshness of blood is also important. During the storage of blood 2,3 DPG reduces, pH reduces, extracellular potassium maximizes, as well as free HgB maximizes. Most blood banks servicing use blood aging less than 7 days old. Preservation of gived blood by anticoagulation is suggested. Anticoagulants usually contain anticoagulant, buffer as well as energy source for erythrocytes (citrate, sodium phosphate, dextrose). Citrate phosphate dextrose (CPD) is the most common preservative applied in transfusions. One unit of whole blood contains 450 ml of donor blood accompanied with 60 ml of CPD. Other additives are not widely applied owing to their possible toxicities (adenine - renal toxicity, mannitol - osmotic diuretic effects as well as dextrose - hyperglycemia).

It should be noted that no information suggests that parents or relatives donating blood is safer than banked blood. Indeed, parents should not give to their child because it reduces the future chance that the parent can bring organs to the child for transplant as well as maternal plasma in postsectionum period usually contains numerous alloantibodies against paternal red blood cells, white blood cells, platelets, as well as HLA antigens.

D. Blood Component from Donation

One unit of blood is consisted of many components. The principal components included red cells, platelets , plasma as well as white cells (rmally not applied) [12]. Before making a transfusion, the physician in charge have to consider that the blood can be or cannot be transfused. Transfusion should be cancelled in cases of failures during production do not pass quality control, outdated as well as delivered to desectionment within more than half an hour. The preparation of blood component poses many steps passing many spinning.

The important blood components include

1. red blood cells

   Red blood cell have to be filtered. Maximized hemolysis with small needles for administration can be seen. It should be noted that fresh blood is less prone to hemolyze as well as pumps do not damage the red cells. Also, blood warmers do not damage the cells. The principal indications include acuted severe anemia as well as chronic anemia with heart as well as lung disease. The dosage depends on the case'age, diseases, symptoms. The advantage of red cell transfusion is maximize of red cell that helps maximize oxygen transportation. Klein et al. said that laboratory assays that indicated failing tissue oxygenation would be ideal to guide the need for transfusion, but none had proved easy, reproducible, as well as sensitive to regional tissue hypoxia [13].

2. Leukocyte depleted (poor) blood (LPB) [14]

   Preparation of LPB is by refrigerated centrifugation or specific leukocyte filter (Sepacell R500 , Imugard IG500 , Pall RC100). The indication includes use for the prevention of transfusion reactive action, alloimmunization to leukocyte antigen, platelet refractoriness as well as CMV infection.

3. Platelet

The principal indication for platelet transfusion is the treatment or prevention of bleeding in profoundly thrombocytopenic cases with bone marrow failure owing to malignancy as well as/or myelosuppressive therapy [15]. The satisfied post transfusion platelet level requires judge for each case. It is usually done with a single transfusion as well as can be transfused as rapidly as the case conditions permits (1 to 2 hours). It should be noted that storage at room temperature is requested but can maximize bacterial risk. At room temperature, platelet can be storage for 5 days. The effect of platelet concentrate storage temperature (4 °C versus room temperature) on platelet adenine nucleotide metabolism was studied by Filip et al. [16]. The results for concentrates stored at room temperature, with a final pH above 6.0, were not inferior to the results for those stored at 4 °C. Filip et al. said that storage at both temperatures was related to conversion of ATP in the metabolic adenine nucleotide pool to hypoxanthine [16].

4. Fresh Frozen Plasma (FFP) [17-18]

FFP is divided from whole blood (WB) within 8 hours as well as immediately frozen in ethanol bath at -4°C or freezer -18°C. The derived FFP should be stored at a temperature of -25 °C or not higher [19]. One unit consists of factor VIII > 0.7 I.U. /ml , red blood cell < 0.6 x 10^9 cells/L , white blood cell < 0.1 x 10^9cells/L , Platelets < 50 x 10^9 cells/L. The thawing can, for example, occur packaged in a plastic bag in a water bath (refresh/clean daily) of 37 °C (with temperature monitoring) [19]. The indication of FFP transfusion include single or multiple coagulation factors defect, reversal of warfarin therapy , plasma exchange therapy for thrombotic thrombocytopenic purpura [20].

5. Cryoprecipitate (Anti-Hemophilia Factor, AHF) [15]

One unit of cryoprecipitate contain factor VIII : C 80 -100 I.U., factor VIII : vWF 40 -70 % , fibrinogen 150 - 300 mg , factor XIII 20 -30 % , plasma 5 -10 ml. The principal indication of cryoprecipitate transfusion include hemophilia A , von Willebrand's disease, obstetric complication , congenital or acquired fibrinogen Defect , factor XIII Defect as well as DIC [20]. However, an important risk of cryoprecipitate is virus contamination. Evatt et al. noted that over a lifetime of treatment (60 years), the cumulative risk of HIV exposure for a person with hemophilia getting monthly infusion of cryoprecipitate prepared from plasma was estimated 2% in the USA as well as 40% in Venezuela [21]. Considering the cumulative risk for transmitting HIV to cases with **hemophilia** through cryoprecipitate treatment, medical care bringrs should carefully evaluate the use of cryoprecipitate in any but emergency conditions or when no virally inactivated outcomes are available. The present trend is changing from from cryoprecipitate to virus-safe high-purity concentrate [22].

6. Cryo - removed plasma (CRP) [15]

One unit of CRP contains plasma volume 200 ml , all stable coagulation factors as well as proteins. The principal indication of CRP transfusion include hemophilia B, replace prothrombin complex (Factor II , VII , IX , X) as well as volume expansion [20].

Summarization on important indication for blood component transfusion [23] is shown in Table 1.

Table 1. Important indications of blood component transfusion

Components	Indications
Whole blood	acute massive blood loss
PRC	severe anemia
platelet	profound thrombocytopenia
FFP	coagulation factor defect, severe coagulopathy
Cryoprecipitate	hypofibrinogenemia, hemophilia A
Cryo - removed plasma	hemophilia B, volume expansion

BLOOD TRANSFUSION FOR NEWBORN

Blood transfusion is a basic practice in medicine. As previously mentioned, it is useful for many pathological conditions. The major indication of blood transfusion is for life saving. There are many kinds of blood transfusions and those types can be applied in neonatology.

A. Whole Blood Transfusion

Whole blood transfusion is extremely indicated in transfusion medicine at present. The transfusion of fresh whole blood (FWB) for trauma-induced coagulopathy is unusual in civilian practice. However, Kauvar et al. said that FWB transfusions were most common when demands for massive transfusions wiped out existing blood supplies [24]. They noted that FWB patients had the highest blood product requirements but fatality did not differ significantly between FWB and non-FWB patients whole or for massively transfused patients [24]. They proposed that FWB might be used in some specific conditions such as during war [24]. Repine et al. proposed that the risk:benefit ratio of FWB transfusion favors its use under extreme circumstances [25] FWB might, at times, be advantageous even when conventional component therapy is available [25]. The FWB transfusion is also restricted used in neonatology

B. Fresh Frozen Plasma

The major indication of FFP is the replacement of plasma, not cellular component. FFP is heavily used in massive transfusion. Although FFP can partially correct abnormal coagulation, a recent systematic review revealed no randomized studies showing clinical benefit [26]. Although the whole risks of FFP is not high, it the least safe blood component, due to immunologic reactions such as allergy/anaphylaxis, transfusion-related acute lung injury (TRALI) and hemolysis due to anti-A or anti-B if transfused across ABO groups [26].

TRALI, an acute syndrome of dyspnoea, hypoxia and pulmonary white-out is present a major cause of transfusion-related death [26]. According to an audit study in a developing country, the use of FFP for volume support in trauma, massive bleeding and burns, routine requests without identified indication in cardiac bypass surgery, and preventive use in the perioperative period can be the basis for suggestions to minimize the inappropriate use of FFP in the future [27].

For newborn, the frequency of specific diseases that might necessitate the administration of FFP differs from that in adults. The plasma levels of many procoagulant factors and important anticoagulants are not higher in newborns than in other age groups, however, healthy newborns show no easy bruising, no increased bleeding during surgery, and excellent wound healing [28]. The good primary hemostasis in newborns despite poor in vitro platelet function seems to be due majorly to a very high von Willebrand factor and the presence of more high-multimeric subunits of von Willebrand factor than later in life [28-29]. Since healthy newborns and young infants have excellent hemostasis, there is absolutely no indication to correct these values to adult's norms prior to invasive procedures by administering FFP [28]. At present, indications for FFP, once used routinely in the support of critically ill infants and children, have become more specific as evolving evidence has confirmed or disproved the efficacy of plasma in various circumstances [29]. FFP is currently indicated to treat the coagulopathies of massive hemorrhage, liver failure and disseminated intravascular coagulation and sepsis [28-29]. Exchange transfusion and extracorporeal membrane oxygenation is additional specific indication for newborns [28]. In congenital clotting factor deficiency, replacement therapy is much more easily administered using a highly specific concentrate [28]. However, when FFP is used to raise the level of the congenitally deficient factor, the huge volume needed to reach sufficiently high plasma levels can commonly be a major problem, therefore, FFP as a replacement therapy in congenital factor deficiency is only indicated when no specific concentrate is available [28].

C. Red Blood Cell Transfusion

Red blood cell transfusion is indicated in cases that need red blood cell such as anemia. Pack red cell (PRC) is the well-known component for red blood cell transfusion. Hematological features indicate that a newborn has a blood volume of 85-125 ml/kg, the fetal hemoglobin is 60-85% and average hemoglobin level in full term infant is 18 gm/dl [30]. It severe neonatal anemia is judged, PRC transfusion should be concerned. Neonatal anemia is an important indication of PRC transfusion. Anemia due to hemorrhage is the most common indication. Hemorrhage can be ante or intra or post natal and it could be external or internal [31]. It could be acute or chronic [31]. Management of acute severe hemorrhage includes packed cell transfusion [31]. However, the red cells transfusions are generally top up exchange transfusions, partial exchange transfusions [30]. Top up- are for investigational losses and correction of mild degrees of anemias, upto to 5-15 ml/kg [30]. They comprise 90% of all neonatal transfusions and are used in not high birth babies in special care units for a maximum of 9-10 episodes [30].

There are also some concerns on the adverse effect of repeated RBC transfusion on newborn. The first concern is about the iron overload. Dani et al. said that gestational age, blood transfusion volume and iron load by transfusions are associated with the risk of occurrence of ROP in infants with a birthweight of less than 1250 grams [32]. Dani et al. also found that plasma non-transferrin bound iron is significantly increased in preterm infants for three hours after PRC transfusion, but this is not associated with significant changes in oxidative stress [33]. Another important concern is the effect on immune system. HLA alloimmunization can be imagined. The leukocyte filter technique has been shown to be effective in preventing HLA alloimmunization and transfusion reactions but the price is rather high [34-35]. For the inverted centrifugation technique, only transfusion reactions were effectively prevented and the HLA alloimmunization continued to develop [35].

D. White Blood Cell Transfusion

White blood cell transfusion is not indicated at present due to the high prevalence of blood borne transfusion. The replacement of white blood cell which is the old indication of buffy coat administration is present replaced by the administration of granulocyte stimulating factor. However, there are some practices of granulocyte transfusions in the cases with severe neonatal sepsis [36-38]. According to a recent Cochrane review, there is inconclusive evidence from randomized control trials to support or refute the routine use of granulocyte transfusions in newborns with sepsis and neutropaenia to reduce fatality and morbidity [36]. Researchers can be encouraged to conduct adequately powered multicentre trials of granulocyte transfusions to clarify their role in newborns with sepsis and neutropaenia [36].

E. Platelet Transfusion

Platelet is a part of cell circulating in the blood stream. Platelet, white blood cell (granulocyte) and red blood cell (erythrocyte) are the three important cellular components of blood. For production of platelet, bone marrow is the factory site. Within the bone marrow, megakaryocytopoiesis involves the commitment of hematopoietic stem cells, and the proliferation, maturation and terminal differentiation of the megakaryocytic progenitors [39]. The major function of platelet is in hemostasis process. Concerning the normal hemostasis process, after the episode of hemorrhage, the vasoconstriction is the first response. Coagulation due to coagulation factors to derive fibrin to weave at the wound occurs and the platelet in the blood stream will be entrapped at that site and result in the wound healing. This process must be balanced by the fibrinolysis system to derive homeostasis. Hence, it can be said that platelet is needed for human beings and defects of platelet, in function or amount, can result in hematological abnormality. Platelet transfusion is a type of blood transfusion. A platelet transfusion is given in the same manner as whole blood. At present, platelet transfusion is widely used in transfusion medicine. There are two important indications for platelet transfusion at present, prophylaxis and therapy. The most important indication for platelet transfusion is the treatment of bleeding episodes in thrombocytopenic patients due to bone marrow aplasia, leukaemia, or chemotherapy of various malignancies [40]. ABO and HLA typing are carried out on donors and recipients [40]. Due to the high polymorphism of the HLA system, it is, however, difficult to find a compatible donor-recipient pair [40]. The indications of important platelet outcomes are discussed. While many advances have been made in platelet transfusion technology, problems remain [41]. These include the short storage life of liquid-stored platelets and the common development of alloantibodies (the refractory state) in patients getting a number of transfusions [41].

Similar to other blood components transfusion, complications due to platelet transfusion is documented. Refractoriness is the most important complication of platelet transfusion therapy, occurring in about 50% of patients getting repeated transfusions [42]. Lack of adequate post-transfusion platelet count increments - platelet refractoriness - is a complication of chronic platelet support shown by 5-15% of chronic platelet recipients [42]. Basically, refractoriness is usually defined as the occurrence of 2-3 post-transfusion platelet count increments, corrected for the patient's size and number of administered platelets, at 10-60 minutes and at 18-24 hours post-transfusion benot high 4,500-5,000 and 2,500 platelets per microliter respectively [43]. Generally, refractoriness is associated with clinical and pharmacological causes in most cases, however, in those cases in which refractoriness is due to immune factors, anti-HLA antibodies are most commonly set [43]. The major causes are HLA alloimmunization and non-immune platelet consumption associated with clinical factors such as septicaemia, DIC and splenomegaly [42]. Initial management of alloimmunized patients who are refractory to platelet transfusions from random donors is the use of HLA-matched platelet transfusions, which improve responses to transfusions in about 65% of patients [42].

In newborn, the platelet transfusion is also indicated for the cases with severe thrombocytopenia. Basically, thrombocytopenia occurs in up to a third of preterm newborns admitted to intensive care units [44]. In these babies, thrombocytopenia typically presents in one of two patterns: early-onset thrombocytopenia occurring within three days of birth and late-onset thrombocytopenia which develops after 72 hours [44].

It is noted that late-onset neonatal thrombocytopenia is usually due to bacterial sepsis or necrotising enterocolitis (NEC); it is often severe, prolonged and requires treatment with platelet transfusions [44]. There is a new concern on platelet transfusion in newborn with NEC. It should be noted that platelet transfusions contain a variety of bioactive factors, including platelet activating factor (PAF), which can augment systemic inflammatory processes [45]. A growing body of evidence that incriminates PAF in the pathogenesis of NEC has emerged over the past few decades from both animal and human data [45]. Both severe thrombocytopenia and multiple platelet transfusions have been associated with increased fatality, but it is admittedly difficult to differentiate between the effects of the underlying disease and the effects, if any, of the platelet transfusions [45].

F. Coagulation Factor Transfusion

Coagulation factor transfusion is an important tool for treatment of the patients with hemophilia [46-47]. The clotting factor can be prepared from the donated blood. The problem on finding of blood donor and donor selection should be mentioned. In addition, the problem of blood borne infection in the present day should be stated. Human immunodeficiency virus (HIV), hepatitis B virus (HBV) and hepatitis C virus (HCV) in the blood supply are the important problematic blood borne transmitted diseases. In general, cryoprecipitate transfusion is the widely used coagulation factor transfusion for the cases with hemophilia [46-48]. According to the study of Evatt et al., over a lifetime of treatment (60 years), the cumulative risk of HIV exposure for a person with hemophilia getting monthly infusion of cryoprecipitate prepared from plasma is significant, 2% in the USA and 40% in Venezuela [49]. Considering the cumulative risk for transmitting HIV to patients with hemophilia through cryoprecipitate treatment, medical care providers should carefully evaluate the use of cryoprecipitate in any but emergency conditions or when no virally inactivated outcomes are available [47]. In more affluent countries, the debate in recent years has focused on the relative merits of plasma versus recombinant outcomes [46]. Coagulation factor concentrates are expensive, and cost-benefit and quality-of-life studies will assume an increasing importance in guiding the selection of outcomes [46]. Looking to the future, genetic engineering brings the potential to create coagulation factors with enhanced properties, such as reduced immunogenicity and prolonged half-life [46].

JAHOVAH WITNESS AND PATIENT'S RIGHTS IN TRANSFUSION MEDICINE

Patient's right is the heart of present medical service. Considering transfusion medicine, a branch of clinical pathology, there is an interesting aspect on patient's right on "Jahovas witness." According to the oaths of the Christian who believe in Jahovas witness principles, receiving blood and blood product is prohibited. Transfusion practice for these patients is an important consideration on patient's rights [47-50]. The aspects for consideration include:

1. Medical practice for Jahovas witness: review on update medical practice [51-52]

   Although there are many scientific conferences and consensus for setting up of clinical practice guideline for the Jahovas witness that bring many new alternative medical practices including artificial blood and bloodless surgery. Can we say that those new medical practices for Jahovas witness follow natural principles and sufficient medical practice?

2. Rights to accept or reject a specific therapeutic option : lesson from medical practice in Jahovas witness cases [47-50,53-54]

   The rights to reject the treatment for the nearly death cases, as in the case of Buddhadasa might be well known [55-56]. However, the rights to accept or reject a specific option, selection, might be a new thing for general physicians. And this challenge the medical practice of many doctors. Although the proposed therapeutic option is the best updated and standard the patients might totally deny. Therefore, what is the role of the physician in charge? A. making an argument, B. following the patient request and saying nothing or C. or? In many countries, the management of Jahovas witness is recommended for special method. Making an argument or trying to pursue the patient may be hopeless and usually bring confrontation. Giving the understanding and knowledge on the risk of the alternative therapy is recommended.

3. Preparation for the fought-to-select medical practice : analysis for the future [47-50]

   Sometimes the medical practice is fought to select by unpredictable factor. Sometimes, the choices are very limited such as those of Jahovas withness. Therefore analysis for alternative, preventive action plan as well as risk estimation is necessary and should be set up to increase the quality of medical service.

4. Medical practice against religious belief : conclusion [56]

   Many accepted standard medical practices at present might be judged as practices that against religious belief. In addition to Jahovas witness, there are also other examples including autopsy examination and preparation for Halal drink and food for the Muslim or preparation for vegetarian food for the strict Mahayana Buddhist vegans. Physician should aware any medical practices that might against the religious belief for these patient. The system as making understanding and giving knowledge on the patient self-selected therapeutic option due to his/her rights must be followed.

REFERENCES

[1] Wiwanitkit V. Blood components in laboratory medicine. *Chula Med J* 2008 (in press)

[2] Marcposes well as J, Gouezec H. Blood transfusion practice. *Transfus Clin Biol.* 2005 Jun;12(2):180-5.

[3] Wiwanitkit V. A study on attitude towards blood donation among people in a rural district, Thailas well as. *Southeast Asian J Trop Med Public Health.* 2000 Sep;31(3):609-11.

[4] Kiefel V. Risk of immunization to blood cells as well as diagnostic as well as therapeutic implications. *Beitr Infusionsther.* 1993;31:44-51.

[5] Perrotta PL, Snyder EL. Non-infectious complicated outcomes of transfusion therapy. *Blood Rev.* 2001 Jun;15(2):69-83.

[6] Blejer JL, Carreras Vescio LA, Salamone HJ. Risk of transfusional-transmitted infections. *Medicina (B Aires).* 2002;62(3):259-78.

[7] Fowler DH. Shared biology of GVHD as well as GVT effects: potential methods of separation. *Crit Rev Oncol Hematol.* 2006 Mar;57(3):225-44.

[8] Bojanic I, Cepulic BG. Transfusion-associated graft-versus-host disease. *Lijec Vjesn.* 2004 Jan-Feb;126(1-2):39-47.

[9] Las well asi EP, de Oliveira JS. Transfusion-associated graft-versus-host disease guideline on gamma irradiation of blood components. *Rev Assoc Med Bras.* 1999 Jul-Sep;45(3):261-72.

[10] Webb DK. Irradiation in the prevention of transfusion associated graft-versus-host disease. *Arch Dis Child.* 1995 Nov;73(5):388-9.

[11] Takaposeshi K. New guideline for transfusion medicine. *Rinsho Byori.* 2006 Dec;54(12):1234-40.

[12] Mooney S. Preparation of blood components. *Probl Vet Med.* 1992 Dec;4(4):594-9.

[13] Klein HG, Spahn DR, Carson JL. Red blood cell transfusion in clinical practice. *Lancet.* 2007 Aug 4;370(9585):415-26.

[14] Lichtiger B, Leparc GF. Leukocyte-poor blood components: issues as well as indications. *Crit Rev Clin Lab Sci.* 1991;28(5-6):387-403.

[15] Wadsworth Center. Guidelines for the transfusion of platelets. Available online at http://www.wadsworth.org/labcert/blood_tissue/platelets.htm

[16] Filip DJ, Eckstein JD, Sibley CA. The effect of platelet concentrate storage temperature on adenine nucleotide metabolism. *Blood.* 1975 Jun;45(6):749-56.

[17] Burnouf T. Modern plasma fractionation. *Transfus Med Rev.* 2007 Apr;21(2):101-17.

[18] Guideline for the use of fresh-frozen plasma. Medical Directors Advisory Committee, National Blood Transfusion Council. *S Afr Med J.* 1998 Oct;88(10):1344-7.

[19] Fresh frozen plasma. Available online at www.sanquin.nl/Sanquin-eng/sqn_outcomes_Blood.nsf/All/Fresh-Frozen-Plasma.html

[20] Williams EF. Current transfusion therapy: indications for basic components. *Clin Lab Sci.* 1994 Jul-Aug;7(4):219-24.

[21] Evatt BL, Austin H, Leon G, Ruiz-Saez A, De Bosch N. Haemophilia therapy: assessing the cumulative risk of HIV exposure by cryoprecipitate. *Haemophilia.* 1999 Sep;5(5):295-300.

[22] Heimburger N. From cryoprecipitate to virus-safe high-purity concentrate. *Semin Thromb Hemost.* 2002 Apr;28 Suppl 1:25-30.

[23] Blood components and blood products. Available online at www.redcross.or.th/extra/blood_seminar_50/files/108_0900-0945.pdf

[24] Kauvar DS, Holcomb JB, Norris GC, Hess JR. Fresh whole blood transfusion: a controversial military practice. *J Trauma.* 2006 Jul;61(1):181-4.

[25] Repine TB, Perkins JG, Kauvar DS, Blackborne L. The use of fresh whole blood in massive transfusion. *J Trauma.* 2006 Jun;60(6 Suppl):S59-69.

[26] MacLennan S, Williamson LM. Risks of fresh frozen plasma and platelets. *J Trauma.* 2006 Jun;60(6 Suppl):S46-50.

[27] Prathiba R, Jayaranee S, Ramesh JC, Lopez CG, Vasanthi N. An audit of fresh frozen plasma usage in a tertiary referral centre in a developing country. *Malays J Pathol.* 2001 Jun;23(1):41-6.

[28] Muntean W. Fresh frozen plasma in the pediatric age group and in congenital coagulation factor deficiency. *Thromb Res.* 2002 Oct 31;107 Suppl 1:S29-32.

[29] Goldenberg NA, Manco-Johnson MJ. Pediatric hemostasis and use of plasma components. *Best Pract Res Clin Haematol.* 2006;19(1):143-55.

[30] Radhakrishnan KM, Chakravarthi S, Pushkala S, Jayaraju J. Component therapy. *Indian J Pediatr.* 2003 Aug;70(8):661-6.

[31] Lokeshwar MR, Dalal R, Manglani M, Shah N. Anemia in newborn. *Indian J Pediatr.* 1998 Sep-Oct;65(5):651-61.

[32] Dani C, Reali MF, Bertini G, Martelli E, Pezzati M, Rubaltelli FF. The role of blood transfusions and iron intake on retinopathy of prematurity. *Early Hum Dev.* 2001 Apr;62(1):57-63.

[33] Dani C, Martelli E, Bertini G, Pezzati M, Rossetti M, Buonocore G, Paffetti P, Rubatelli FF. Effect of blood transfusions on oxidative stress in preterm infants. *Arch Dis Child Fetal Neonatal Ed.* 2004 Sep;89(5):F408-11.

[34] Chuansumrit A, Nathalang O, Wangruansathit S, Hathirat P, Chiewsilp P, Isarangura P. HLA alloimmunization in patientsgettingmultitransfusions of red blood cells. *Southeast Asian J Trop Med Public Health.* 2001 Jun;32(2):419-24.

[35] Tan KK, Lee WS, Liaw LC, Oh A. A prospective study on the use of leucocyte-filters in reducing blood transfusion reactions in multi-transfused thalassemic children. *Singapore Med J.* 1993 Apr;34(2):109-11.

[36] Mohan P, Brocklehurst P. Granulocyte transfusions for neonates with confirmed or suspected sepsis and neutropaenia. *Cochrane Database Syst Rev* 2003;(4):CD003956.

[37] Baley JE, Stork EK, Warkentin PI, Shurin SB. Buffy coat transfusions in neutropenic neonates with presumed sepsis: a prospective, randomized trial. *Pediatrics. 1987 Nov;80(5):712-20.*

[38] Wheeler JG, Chauvenet AR, Johnson CA, Block SM, Dillard R, Abramson JS. Buffy coat transfusions in neonates with sepsis and neutrophil storage pool depletion. *Pediatrics.* 1987 Mar;79(3):422-5.

[39] Deutsch VR, Tomer A. Megakaryocyte development and platelet production. *Br J Haematol.* 2006 Jul 20;

[40] Seidl S, Kilp M. The current status of platelet and granulocyte transfusions. *Haematologia (Budap).* 1980;13(1-4):145-54.

[41] Kelton JG, Blajchman MA. Platelet transfusions. *Can Med Assoc J.* 1979 Nov 17;121(10):1353-8.

[42] Murphy MF, Waters AH. Clinical aspects of platelet transfusions. *Blood Coagul Fibrinolysis.* 1991 Apr;2(2):389-96.

[43] Rubella P. A mini-review on platelet refractoriness. *Haematologica.* 2005 Feb;90(2):247-53.

[44] Chakravorty S, Murray N, Roberts I. Neonatal thrombocytopenia. *Early Hum Dev.* 2005 Jan;81(1):35-41.

[45] Fernandes CJ, O'Donovan DJ. Platelet transfusions in infants with necrotizing enterocolitis. *Curr Hematol Rep.* 2006 Mar;5(1):76-81.

[46] Giangrande PL. Blood products for hemophilia: past, present and future. *BioDrugs.* 2004;18(4):225-34.

[47] Aguilera P. Blood transfusions in Jehovah's witnesses. *Rev Med Chil.* 1993;121:447-51.

[48] McDonald RT, Wren LT. Blood, the Jehovah Witness and the physician. *Ariz Med.* 1967;24:969-73.

[49] Cagne C. Knowing and understanding a Jehovah Witness patient. *Part two. Rev Infirm.* 1995;(1):57-62.

[50] Loriau J, Manaouil C, Montpellier D, Graser M, Jarde O. Surgery and transfusion in Jehovah's witness patient. Medical legal review. *Ann Chir.* 2004;129:263-8.

[51] Chua R, Tham KF. Will "no blood" kill Jehovah Witnesses? *Singapore Med J.* 2006;47:994-1001.

[52] Phaosavasdi S, Wilde H, Pruksapong C, Tannirandorn Y. Ethics and care of the terminally ill. *J Med Assoc Thai*. 1998;81:468-71.

[53] Phaosavasdi S, Thamkhantho M, Uerpairojkit B, Pruksapong C, Kanjanapitak A. Searching for medical ethics in Dharma conversation. *J Med Assoc Thai.* 2005;88:440-1.

[54] Woolley S. Jehovah's Witnesses in the emergency department: what are their rights? *Emerg Med J*. 2005;22:869-71.

[55] McInroy A. Blood transfusion and Jehovah's Witnesses: the legal and ethical issues. *Br J Nurs*. 2005;14:270-4.

[56] Bourgeois M, Khaleff M, Labrousse D. A religious sect, its mental ill patients, its physician and its psychiatrists. *Ann Med Psychol (Paris)*. 1975;1:160-7.

Chapter IX

PHOTOTHERAPY

INTRODUCTION

Light is a basic thing that human beings know. Light is mainly from the sun. Electricity can also provide light. Therapy by light is also a medical concept. Since light poses energy therefore it might be used for treatment. In this chapter, the author will present the topic on phototherapy. Main kinds of application, photodynamic therapy and classical phototherapy for newborn will be discussed.

PHOTODYNAMIC THERAPY

A. What is Photodynamic Therapy?

Photodynamic therapy (PDT) is a novel medical therapy making used of a non-toxic dye termed a photosensitizer (PS) together with low intensity visible light, which, in the presence of oxygen, generate cytotoxic species [1]. PS can be targeted to its destination cell or tissue and, in addition, the irradiation can be spatially confined to the lesion giving PDT the advantage of increased doubled selectivity [1]. In therapy, PDT can lead to photochemical tissue destruction or immunomodulation [2]. The greatest disadvantage of systemic administration of photosensitizers is cutaneous photosensitization of the patients, which can presist for some months [2].

Presently, PDT is an approved treatment for several types of tumors and certain benign diseases. Physiologically, light-activation of the photosensitizer in the presence of molecular oxygen, which accumulates in cancer tissues, brings the local production of reactive oxygen species that kill the tumor cells [3]. Hendrickx *et al.* reported that hypericin-mediated PDT of human cancer cells led to up-regulation of the inducible cyclooxygenase-2 (COX-2) enzyme and the subsequent release of PGE2 [4]. They noted that the combination of PDT with pyridinyl imidazole inhibitors of p38 MAPK might improve the therapeutic efficacy of PDT by blocking COX-2 up-regulation, which contributed to tumor growth by the release of growth- and pro-angiogenic factors, as well as by sensitizing cancer cells to apoptosis [4].Agostinis *et al.* noted that mitochondria were central coordinators of the mechanisms by which PDT induced apoptosis in the target cells [3].Agostinis *et al.* also noted that concomitant to the permeabilization of the outer mitochondrial membrane, which led to the release of several apoptogenic factors in the cytosol and to the activation of effector caspases, regulatory signaling pathways were activated in a photosensitizer, PDT dose and cell-dependent fashion [3]. They proposed that signaling pathways regulated by members of mitogen activated protein kinases and their downstream targets, such as cyclooxygenase-2, appeared to critically modulate cancer cell sensitivity to PDT [3]. Almeida *et al.* said that activation of phospholipases, changes in ceramide metabolism, a rise in the cytosolic free Ca2+ concentration, stimulation of nitric oxide synthase (NOS), changes in protein phosphorylation and alterations in the activity of transcription factors and on gene expression had all been observed in PDT-treated cells [5]. Ali *et al.* said that loss of mitochondrial transmembrane potential, release of cytochrome c, involvement of caspases-8 and -3 and the status caspase-3 specific substrate PARP, were evaluated in PDT treated tumor cells [6]. They also noted that caspase-3 plays an important role in induced apoptosis [6]. Components of the mechanism whereby PDT causes cells to undergo apoptosis are becoming understood, as are the influences of several signal transduction pathways on the response [7]. Finally, Almeida *et al.* said that understanding the signaling mechanisms in PDT might provide means to modulate the PDT effects at the molecular level and potentiate its antitumor effectiveness [5].

PDT is presently accepted as a new integrative cancer therapy [8]. Indeed, PDT is widely applied for gastrointestinal diseases including obstructing oesophageal cancer, early-stage oesophageal cancer, Barrett's esophagus, hilar cholangiocarcinoma, stomach-, colon- and pancreatic cancer [9]. An example on application for cholangiocarcinoma will be hereby presented.

B. Cholangiocarcinoma, a Tropical Carcinoma

Cholangiocarcinoma is an important tropical carcinoma. It is an uncommon malignant tumor arising from the biliary epithelium. The incidence of this cancer significantly increases with age and usually affects individuals in their 6th or 7th decade of life [10]. Presently, cholangiocarcinoma is a common cancer among the people in Southeast Asia, with the world highest prevalence at the northeastern Thailand and Laos [11]. Unfortunately, most of the patients with cholangiocarcinoma presented to the physicians with advance diseases resulting in several complications and highly fatal outcomes [12]. The most commonly observed clinical symptoms and signs were fever, abdominal pain, malaise and weakness [12]. Wiwanitkit said that most of cholangiocarcinoma are at distal extrahepatic following by seven perihilar and intrahepatic [12]. Wiwanitkit also noted that almost half of the patients presented with other pathological conditions, resulting from acute biliary tract obstruction and ascites [12]. Of those complications, acute cholangitis is one of the common complications of cholangiocarcioma [13]. Wiwanitkit proposed that the pathogens detected were similar in cases of cholangitis alone and cholangiocarcinoma [12].

Concerning the laboratory finding in this tumor, a significant increase in serum bilirubin and marked elevation of serum alkaline phosphatase (ALP) can be seen. Wiwanitkit said that high serum ALP levels in hospitalized patients were commonly found in three major groups having obstructive biliary diseases and cholangiocarcionoma was the most common cancer with a marked elevation of serum ALP [14]. Paritpokee *et al.* noted that the fast liver isoenzyme could be a useful marker in diagnosis of malignant extrahepatic obstruction, cholangiocarcinoma [15]. As already mentioned, most of the patients with this cancer usually visit the physician with the late stage of disease and their prognosis is usually grave. The prognosis of perihilar cholangiocarcinoma (CC) is limited by tumor spread along the biliary tree leading to refractory obstructive cholestasis, cholangitis, and liver failure [10]. Prognosis of cholangiocarcinomas is dismal, although five-year survival rates for these cancers have improved due to the recent progress in surgery and adjuvant oncological therapy [16].

The first-line imaging investigation is ultrasonography, which usually detects dilatation of the bile ducts, but more rarely the tumor itself [16]. Classically, endoscopic retrograde cholangiopancreatography (ERCP), the gold standard investigation in case of obstructive jaundice, is also recommended [16]. Concerning treatment, surgical procedure is the widely used method for cholangiocarcinoma therapy [17]. Acalovschi said that all patients who do not have unequivocal cholangiographic and angiographic signs of unresectability should undergo surgery, in order to benefit of a possible tumor resection [16]. Acalovschi noted that the radical surgical procedures relieved the obstruction and jaundice by resecting the tumor [16]. Palliation with biliary endoprostheses results in median survival times between 4 and 6 months for non-resectable cholangiocarcinoma [10]. In advance cases, the palliative, surgical or endoscopic, procedures cure the jaundice, but cannot remove the tumor [16]. Primary prevention for this cancer is proposed to be more useful than therapy. The major risk factor for this cancer in the endemic area is believed to be exposure to liver fluke, *Opisthorchis viverrini*, in insufficiently cooked traditional foods [12]. Other risk factors include primary sclerosing cholangitis (PSC) and choledochal cysts. As this cancer is still endemic in Southeast Asia, continuous prevention and surveillance of this public health problem are necessary for this region.

C. Application of Photodynamic Therapy in Cholangiocarcinoma

General Introduction

As previously mentioned, PDT can be applied in cholangiocarcinoma [18-19]. Generally, the therapeutic principle of resecting liver tumors, applies to both primary and secondary types of liver abnormal tumors [20]. Unfortunately many patients with many liver lesions, especially cholangiocarcinoma, are inoperable due to technical difficulties or comorbidity [20]. Although surgical resection offers the only hope for cure, most patients are found to have unresectable disease on initial presentation and have an extremely grim prognosis and this has brought an emphasis on the role of palliative care, with relief of biliary obstruction, in the management of these affected cases [21]. This also stimulated the development of ablation methods, including PDT [20-22].

Indeed, surgical bypass was once the primary means of palliation of obstructive jaundice in patients with unresectable cholangiocarcinoma but in the recent years has been superseded by less invasive and less morbid nonsurgical procedures such as endoscopic and percutaneous biliary stent placement [21]. Newer modalities of palliation such as endoscopic delivery of photodynamic therapy and high-intensity ultrasound therapy are new emerging nonsurgical modalities that may result in improved survival and may be a future hope as an adjunctive therapy to surgical resection [21]. Ortner said that prognosis of nonresectable cholangiocarcinoma is not good, and in Bismuth type III and IV tumors relief of jaundice was seldom achieved, despite successful endoprosthesis insertion and additional photodynamic therapy seems to be a promising new approach to these tumors [23]. Wong Kee Song *et al.* said that despite their relatively localized nature, the therapy for surgically unresectable cholangiocarcinomas had been largely unsuccessful and PDT was a promising technique for both curative and palliative treatment of this malignancy [24]. They recently performed an interesting to compare the effectiveness of a potential new photosensitizer, mono-l-aspartyl chlorin e6 (NPe6) with that of a traditional drug, hematoporphyrin derivative (HpD), in PDT administered to a human cholangiocarcinoma model [24]. According to this study, they concluded that PDT with HpD or NPe6 was effective inducing tumor regression in the cholangiocarcinoma model and NPe6 appeared to induce greater tumor regression than HpD, with decreased tumor regrowth and duration of cutaneous photosensitization [24].Berr said that PDT with porfimer and laser light of 630 nm provides tumoricidal tissue penetration to a depth of only 4 to 4.5 mm that does not eradicate most tumors [10]. Oertel *et al.* said that PDT of bile duct cancer using HpD and laser light of 630 nm wavelength was confined to a tumouricidal tissue penetration of 4 mm, which might be doubled with laser light between 700 and 800 nm [25]. Oertel *et al.* recently investigated the photosensitising properties of a novel bacteriochlorine, tetrakis-pyridyl-tetrahydroporphyrin tosylat (THP) with high absorption at 763 nm [25]. In their study, two biliary cancer cell lines (BDC, GBC) were incubated with HPD or THP to assess cellular uptake kinetics, dark cytotoxicity, and photodynamic cytotoxicity (laser light exposure 1-20 J/cm2) [25]. Oertel *et al.* found that THP induced tumour-selective phototoxicity in the cholangiocarcinoma model and concluded that this novel bacteriochlorine THP exhibited photosensitiser properties in biliary tract cancer cells in vitro and in vivo and could achieve deep tumouricidal tissue penetration due to photoactivation at 763 nm [25]. Ortner said that encouraging results from trials of photodynamic therapy in nonresectable cholangiocarcinoma suggested considerable promise for this new palliative treatment modality [26]. Gerhardt et al. said that pilot studies showed relief of jaundice, mainly because of opening of the intrahepatic ducts and improvements in quality of life indices [22]. They said that survival time seems to be long; however, randomized studies are necessary to confirm these results [22]. However, Ortner said that the apparent benefit of photodynamic therapy on survival, jaundice, and quality of life must be confirmed [26]. Here, the reports on these outcomes of PDT in cholangiocarcinoma are summarized and present.

Survival after PDT

In 2004, Berr noted that tumor ablation with PDT combined with biliary stenting reduces cholestasis and significantly improves median survival time to 11.5 to 16.2 months [10]. Berr also said that time to progression lasted approximately 6 months indicating that PDT was required twice annually [10]. In 2003, Ortner *et al.* performed a prospective, open-label, randomized, multicenter study with a group sequential design compared PDT in addition to stenting (group A) with stenting alone (group B) in patients with cholangiocarcinoma [27]. According to this study, PDT resulted in prolongation of survival [27]. Ortner *et al.* said that PDT, given in addition to best supportive care, undoubtedly improved survival in patients with cholangiocarcinoma and PDT proved to be so superior to simple stenting treatment [27]. Ortner *et al.* performed another interesting study in 9 patients with advanced nonresectable cholangiocarcinomas Bismuth type III and IV, who showed no sufficient drainage (bilirubin decrease <50%) [28]. In this study, after endoscopic stent insertion, all patient were underwent photodynamic therapy [28]. Ortner *et al.* found that thirty-day mortality was 0%, and median survival time was 439 days [28]. Ortner concluded that survival time in cholangiocarcinoma patients after PDT seemed to be prolonged [28-29]. However, there are also some studies indicating that the patients with PDT do not have significantly difference in survival comparing to those without [30].

Jaundice after PDT

Dumoulin *et al.* noted that the combination of PDT and biliary drainage by plastic endoprosthesis insertion has produced promising results in the treatment of nonresectable cholangiocarcinoma [30]. They performed a study to evaluate the feasibility and efficacy of intraductal PDT therapy with subsequent biliary drainage by metal stent insertion in 24 patients [30]. In this study, a significant decrease in serum bilirubin was noted in all patients [30]. Ortner *et al.* said that improved biliary drainage could be derived after PDT [27]. They also noted for significant lowering of hyperbilirubinemia after PDT in addition to stenting comparing to stenting alone [27]. Ortner *et al.* noted that serum bilirubin levels significantly declined after PDT and showed no significant increase during the two monthly follow-ups [28]. They noted that PDT was effective in restoring biliary drainage [28]. Ortner summarized that a remarkable reduction of bile duct stenosis and bilirubin decrease in cholangiocarcinoma patients could be seen after PDT [29]. Rumalla *et al.* said that PDT provided effective relief from biliary obstruction in advanced cholangiocarcinoma [31]. They also noted that PDT for cholangiocarcinoma was safe and technically feasible with a preloaded biliary catheter and a monorail technique for catheter positioning [31]. Ortner noted that PDT was well tolerated, with only few specific side-effects [32]. Reported complications due to PDT include acute cholangitis and skin phototoxicity [31]. However, Wiedmann *et al.* said that PDT for cholangiocarcinoma was a low-risk procedure with efficient selective destruction of the bile duct tumor [33].

Table 1. Reports on photodynamic therapy for other important cancers

Authors	Details
Solár et al. [36]	Solár et al. reported on erythropoietin inhibits apoptosis induced by photodynamic therapy in ovarian cancer cells [36].
Patel et al. [37]	Patel et al. reported on motexafin lutetium-photodynamic therapy of prostate cancer [37].
Milla et al. [38]	Milla et al. reported on pharmacokinetic, toxicological and phototherapeutic studies of phthalocyanine ZnPcCF(3) [38].
Park et al. [39]	Park et al. reported on paclitaxel augments cytotoxic effect of photodynamic therapy using verteporfin in gastric and bile duct cancer cells [39]
Olejek et al. [40]	Olejek et al. reported on photodynamic therapy in vulvar intraepithelial neoplasia [40].
Peng et al. [41]	Peng et al. reported on self-assembled star-shaped chlorin-core poly(varepsilon-caprolactone)-poly(ethylene glycol) diblock copolymer micelles for dual chemo-photodynamic therapies [41].
Stephan et al. [42]	Stephan et al. reported on Photodynamic therapy in retinoblastoma: effects of verteporfin on retinoblastoma cell line [42].
Prasad et al. [43]	Prasad et al. reported on correlation of histology with biomarker status after photodynamic therapy in Barrett esophagus [43]. Prasad concluded that histologic downgrading of dysplasia after photodynamic therapy was associated with the loss of biomarkers that have been associated with progression of neoplasia in Barrett esophagus [43].
Saw et al. [44]	Saw et al. reported on potentiation of the photodynamic action of hypericin [44]. Saw et al. said that hypericin photodynamic diagnosis and hypericin photodynamic therapy could be enhanced and optimized with the right combination of light dosimetry and drug dose in an effective formulation containing a suitable adjuvant [44]. Saw et al. also wrote that hyperoxygenation and hyperthermia could also be used to further enhance the efficacy of hypericin photodynamic therapy [44].
Bhuvaneswari et al. [45]	Bhuvaneswari et al. reported on molecular profiling of angiogenesis in hypericin mediated photodynamic therapy [45]. Bhuvaneswari et al. concluded that long drug light interval hypericin photodynamic therapy induced upregulation of angiogenic proteins [45]. They also noted that differential expression of genes involved in the angiogenesis pathway was observed in the various groups treated with hypericin photodynamic therapy [45].
Matin et al. [46]	Matin et al. reported on a pilot trial of vascular targeted photodynamic therapy for renal tissue [46]. Matin et al. provided the initial proof of principle that justifies further preclinical investigation of vascular targeted photodynamic therapy for renal malignancies [46].
Miura et al. [47]	Miura et al. reported on a new technique for improving visualization of mucosal lesions during endoscopic photodynamic therapy [47].
Sutedja [48]	Sutedja reported on photodynamic therapy in advanced tracheobronchial cancers [48].
Kato et al. [49]	Kato et al. concluded that photodynamic therapy for early stage lung cancer was cost-effective [49].
Okunaka et al. [50]	Okunaka et al. reported on lung cancers treated with photodynamic therapy and surgery [50]. Okunaka et al. concluded that photodynamic therapy as preoperative laser irradiation could contribute to the management of advanced lung malignancy [50].
McCaughan [51]	McCaughan reported on photodynamic therapy for obstructive esophageal malignancies [51]. McCaughan concluded that photodynamic therapy for esophageal carcinoma caused minimal complications and procedure related mortality and complete obstruction could be relieved by the end of the photodynamic therapy endoscopy [51].
Miura et al. [52]	Miura et al. reported on progress of photodynamic therapy in gastric cancer [52].
MacCormack [53]	MacCormack discussed on photodynamic therapy in dermatology [53].

Table 2. Reports on phototherapy for neonatal jaundice

Authors	Details
Ostrow et al. [54]	Ostrow et al. reported on phototherapy for neonatal jaundice [54].
Boo and Chew [55]	Boo and Chew reported on a randomised control trial of clingfilm for prevention of hypothermia in term infants during phototherapy [55].
Djokomuljanto et al. [56]	Djokomuljanto et al. reported that efficacy of phototherapy for neonatal jaundice is increased by the use of low-cost white reflecting curtains [56]. They noted that Hanging white curtains around phototherapy units significantly maximized efficacy of phototherapy in the treatment of neonatal jaundice without evidence of increased adverse effects [56].
Yaseen et al. [57]	Yaseen et al. said that prophylactic phototherapy was associated with a significant reduction of total serum bilirubin in the first 48 hours of life but not later on [57].
Bader et al. [58]	Bader et al. reported on effect of phototherapy on cardiorespiratory activity during sleep in neonates with physiologic jaundice [58]. Bader et al. found that phototherapy could affect the cardiorespiratory activity during active sleep but not during quiet sleep in term infants with physiologic jaundice [58].
Murki et al. [59]	Murki et al. reported on a randomized, triple-blind, placebo-controlled trial of prophylactic oral phenobarbital to reduce the need for phototherapy in G6PD-deficient neonates [59]. Murki et al. concluded that prophylactic oral phenobarbital did not reduce the need for phototherapy or exchange transfusions in G6PD-deficient neonates [59].
Mohammadzadeh et al. [60]	Mohammadzadeh et al. reported on supine versus turning position on bilirubin level during phototherapy in healthy term jaundiced neonates [60].
Turan et al. [61]	Turan et al. reported on impact of phototherapy on vasoactive mediators [61]. Turan et al. found that the group of the neonates close or remote phototherapy caused some body temperature, heart rate and blood pressure changes that were not clinically significant and did not result in increased levels of vasoactive mediators [61].

Quality of Life after PDT

Berr noted that PDT costed less and enhances quality of life and survival time as compared with chemotherapy [10]. Ortner *et al.* found that quality of life after PDT in addition to stenting was significant higher than stenting alone [27]. Ortner *et al.* noted that qality of life indices improved dramatically and remained stable after PDT [28]. They concluded that there were clear evidences that PDT improved quality of life in the patients with cholangiocarcinoma [28]. Many similar studies [31-32] also showed similar results in quality of life improvement in cholangiocarcinoma patients after PDT. Orntner concluded that PDT in non-resectable cholangiocarcinoma had considerable benefit on survival with a good quality of life [32]. Berr suggested that PDT should be offered as part of the palliative treatment of CC in hepatobiliary referral centers [10].

In summary, most previous reports confirmed the advantage of PDT in cholangiocarcinoma. Improvements of survival period, biliary duct obstruction and quality of life are mentioned [34]. By PDT it also seems probable to achieve an improvement of the prognosis in cholangiocarcinoma [35]. As the result of PDT, improvement of quality of life by removing the jaundice, and its important consequence pruritus, is proper for the aim of palliative therapy of malignant bile duct stenosis [35]. Wiedmann *et al.* said that this was of great importance in those cholangiocarcinoma patients with short life expectancy and PDT should therefore be offered to all patients with non resectable cholangiocarcinoma [33]. However, before initiating PDT or any other palliative measure, a proper staging and a surgical consultation is needed to avoid missing a curative surgical option [33].

CLASSICAL PHOTOTHERAPY FOR NEWBORN

Neonatal jaundice is an important problem in medicine. Around 80 per cent of preterm infants develop hyperbilirubinaemia and presented jaundice. Concerning the cause, hyperbilirubinemia can be pre-hepatic, hepatic or post-hepatic originated. A common serious cause is usually due to neonatal hemolytic episode, a case of pre-hepatic hyperbilirubinemia. One of the most fatal unwanted of neonatal jaundice is kernicterus. Historically, the presence of yellow staining and damage to the brain caused by unconjugated bilirubin Neonatal jaundice is an important problem that requires proper management. Exchange transfusion might be used. Administration of Phenobarbital is another alternative. However, one of the most widely used methods is the phototherapy. This is classical practice in many neonatal units. Important interesting reports on this topic will be presented in Table 2.

REFERENCES

[1] Demidova TN, Hamblin MR. Photodynamic therapy targeted to pathogens. *Int J Immunopathol Pharmacol* 2004;17:245-54

[2] Dragieva G, Scharer L, Dummer R, Kempf W. Photodynamic therapy--a new treatment option for epithelial malignancies of the skin. *Onkologie* 2004;27:407-11

[3] Agostinis P, Buytaert E, Breyssens H, Hendrickx N. Regulatory pathways in photodynamic therapy induced apoptosis. *Photochem Photobiol Sci* 2004;3:721-9

[4] Hendrickx N, Volanti C, Moens U, Seternes OM, de Witte P, Vandenheede JR, Piette J, Agostinis P. Up-regulation of cyclooxygenase-2 and apoptosis resistance by p38 MAPK in hypericin-mediated photodynamic therapy of human cancer cells. *J Biol Chem* 2003;278:52231-9

[5] Almeida RD, Manadas BJ, Carvalho AP, Duarte CB. Intracellular signaling mechanisms in photodynamic therapy. *Biochim Biophys Acta.* 2004;1704:59-86

[6] Ali SM, Chee SK, Yuen GY, Olivo M. Photodynamic therapy induced Fas-mediated apoptosis in human carcinoma cells. *Int J Mol Med* 2002;9:257-70

[7] Oleinick NL, Morris RL, Belichenko I. The role of apoptosis in response to photodynamic therapy: what, where, why, and how. *Photochem Photobiol Sci* 2002;1:1-21

[8] Paleev NR, Karandashov VI, Petukhov EB, Diasamidze IuS. Phototherapy and its place in modern medicine. *Vestn Ross Akad Med Nauk* 2004;(7):15-9

[9] Wiedmann MW, Caca K. General principles of photodynamic therapy (PDT) and gastrointestinal applications. *Curr Pharm Biotechnol.* 2004 Aug;5(4):397-408
[10] Berr F. Photodynamic therapy for cholangiocarcinoma. *Semin Liver Dis.* 2004 May;24(2):177-87.
[11] Kullavanijaya P, Tangkijvanich P, Poovorawan Y. Current status of infection-related gastrointestinal and hepatobiliary diseases in Thailand. *Southeast Asian J Trop Med Public Health* 1999; 30: 96-105.
[12] Wiwanitkit V. Clinical findings among 62 Thais with cholangiocarcinoma. *Trop Med Int Health.* 2003 Mar;8(3):228-30.
[13] Nauta RJ. Cholangitis, hemobilia, and cholangiocarcinoma. Management of a fistula between an obstructed right hepatic duct and the portal vein. *Cancer* 1989; 64: 542-6.
[14] Wiwanitkit V. High serum alkaline phosphatase levels, a study in 181 Thai adult hospitalized patients. *BMC Fam Pract* 2001;2:2
[15] Paritpokee N, Tangkijvanich P, Teerasaksilp S, Wiwanitkit V, Lertmaharit S, Tosukhowong P. Fast liver alkaline phosphatase isoenzyme in diagnosis of malignant biliary obstruction. *J Med Assoc Thai* 1999;82:1241-6
[16] Acalovschi M. Cholangiocarcinoma: risk factors, diagnosis and management. *Rom J Intern Med* 2004;42:41-58
[17] Goldberg MJ. Cholangiocarcinoma. *Dis Mon* 2004;50:540-4
[18] Gores GJ. A spotlight on cholangiocarcinoma. *Gastroenterology* 2003;125:1536-8
[19] Burdick JS, Magee D, Miller G, Wright KB. Biliary photodynamic therapy alternative delivery technique. *Endoscopy* 2000;32:S63
[20] Zuber-Jerger I, Geissler M, Spangenberg HC, Mohr L, Weizsacker F, Blum HE. Local ablation of malignant lesions of the liver - potential applications and limitations of the different methods. *Z Gastroenterol* 2004;42:31-8
[21] Abu-Hamda EM, Baron TH. Endoscopic management of cholangiocarcinoma. *Semin Liver Dis* 2004;24:165-75
[22] Gerhardt T, Mey U, Sauerbruch T, Dumoulin FL. Palliative therapy of inoperable cholangiocarcinoma. *Dtsch Med Wochenschr* 2002;127:1835-9
[23] Ortner MA. Photodynamic therapy of cholangiocarcinoma cancer. *Gastrointest Endosc Clin N Am* 2000;10:481-6
[24] Wong Kee Song LM, Wang KK, Zinsmeister AR. Mono-L-aspartyl chlorin e6 (NPe6) and hematoporphyrin derivative (HpD) in photodynamic therapy administered to a human cholangiocarcinoma model. *Cancer* 1998;82:421-7
[25] Oertel M, Schastak SI, Tannapfel A, Hermann R, Sack U, Mossner J, Berr F. Novel bacteriochlorine for high tissue-penetration: photodynamic properties in human biliary tract cancer cells in vitro and in a mouse tumour model. *J Photochem Photobiol B* 2003;71:1-10
[26] Ortner M. Photodynamic therapy in the biliary tract. Curr Gastroenterol Rep 2001;3:154-9
[27] Ortner ME, Caca K, Berr F, Liebetruth J, Mansmann U, Huster D, Voderholzer W, Schachschal G, Mossner J, Lochs H. Successful photodynamic therapy for nonresectable cholangiocarcinoma: a randomized prospective study. *Gastroenterology* 2003;125:1355-63

[28] Ortner MA, Liebetruth J, Schreiber S, Hanft M, Wruck U, Fusco V, Muller JM, Hortnagl H, Lochs H. Photodynamic therapy of nonresectable cholangiocarcinoma. *Gastroenterology* 1998;114:536-42

[29] Ortner M. Photodynamic therapy for cholangiocarcinoma. *J Hepatobiliary Pancreat Surg* 2001;8:137-9

[30] Dumoulin FL, Gerhardt T, Fuchs S, Scheurlen C, Neubrand M, Layer G, Sauerbruch T. Phase II study of photodynamic therapy and metal stent as palliative treatment for nonresectable hilar cholangiocarcinoma. *Gastrointest Endosc* 2003;57:860-7

[31] Rumalla A, Baron TH, Wang KK, Gores GJ, Stadheim LM, de Groen PC. Endoscopic application of photodynamic therapy for cholangiocarcinoma. *Gastrointest Endosc* 2001;53:500-4

[32] Ortner MA. Photodynamic therapy in cholangiocarcinomas. *Best Pract Res Clin Gastroenterol* 2004;18:147-54\

[33] Wiedmann M, Caca K, Berr F, Schiefke I, Tannapfel A, Wittekind C, Mossner J, Hauss J, Witzigmann H. Neoadjuvant photodynamic therapy as a new approach to treating hilar cholangiocarcinoma: a phase II pilot study. *Cancer* 2003;97:2783-90

[34] Terruzzi V, Minoli G. Photodynamic therapy of nenresectable cholangiocarcinoma. *Gastrointest Endosc* 1999; 50:727-8

[35] Hartmann D, Jakobs R, Schilling D, Riemann JF. Endoscopic and radiological interventional therapy of benign and malignant bile duct stenoses. *Zentralbl Chir* 2003;128:936-43.

[36] Solár P, Koval J, Mikes J, Kleban J, Solárová Z, Lazúr J, Hodorová I, Fedorocko P, Sytkowski AJ. Erythropoietin inhibits apoptosis induced by photodynamic therapy in ovarian cancer cells. *Mol Cancer Ther*. 2008 Aug 6. [Epub ahead of print]

[37] Patel H, Mick R, Finlay J, Zhu TC, Rickter E, Cengel KA, Malkowicz SB, Hahn SM, Busch TM. Motexafin lutetium-photodynamic therapy of prostate cancer: short- and long-term effects on prostate-specific antigen. *Clin Cancer Res*. 2008 Aug 1;14(15):4869-76.

[38] Milla LN, Yslas EI, Cabral A, Durantini EN, Romanini S, Rivarola V, Bertuzzi M. Pharmacokinetic, toxicological and phototherapeutic studies of phthalocyanine ZnPcCF(3). *Biomed Pharmacother*. 2008 Mar 14. [Epub ahead of print]

[39] Park S, Hong SP, Oh TY, Bang S, Chung JB, Song SY. Paclitaxel augments cytotoxic effect of photodynamic therapy using verteporfin in gastric and bile duct cancer cells. *Photochem Photobiol Sci*. 2008 Jul;7(7):769-74.

[40] Olejek A, Kozak-Darmas I, Biniszkiewicz T, Kellas-Sleczka S, Sieroń A. Photodynamic therapy in vulvar intraepithelial neoplasia. *Ginekol Pol*. 2008 Apr;79(4):276-80.

[41] Peng CL, Shieh MJ, Tsai MH, Chang CC, Lai PS. Self-assembled star-shaped chlorin-core poly(varepsilon-caprolactone)-poly(ethylene glycol) diblock copolymer micelles for dual chemo-photodynamic therapies. *Biomaterials*. 2008 Sep;29(26):3599-608.

[42] Stephan H, Boeloeni R, Eggert A, Bornfeld N, Schueler A. Photodynamic therapy in retinoblastoma: effects of verteporfin on retinoblastoma cell lines. *Invest Ophthalmol Vis Sci*. 2008 Jul;49(7):3158-63.

[43] Prasad GA, Wang KK, Halling KC, Buttar NS, Wongkeesong LM, Zinsmeister AR, Brankley SM, Westra WM, Lutzke LS, Borkenhagen LS, Dunagan K. Correlation of histology with biomarker status after photodynamic therapy in Barrett esophagus. *Cancer.* 2008 Aug 1;113(3):470-6.

[44] Saw CL, Heng PW, Olivo M. Potentiation of the photodynamic action of hypericin. *J Environ Pathol Toxicol Oncol.* 2008;27(1):23-33.

[45] Bhuvaneswari R, Gan YY, Lucky SS, Chin WW, Ali SM, Soo KC, Olivo M. Molecular profiling of angiogenesis in hypericin mediated photodynamic therapy. *Mol Cancer.* 2008 Jun 13;7:56.

[46] Matin SF, Tinkey PT, Borne AT, Stephens LC, Sherz A, Swanson DA. A pilot trial of vascular targeted photodynamic therapy for renal tissue. *J Urol.* 2008 Jul;180(1):338-42.

[47] Mimura S, Narahara H, Murakami T, Otani T, Hirano T, Suzuki K. A new technique for improving visualization of mucosal lesions during endoscopic photodynamic therapy. *Diagn Ther Endosc.* 2000;6(4):147-52.

[48] Sutedja TG. Photodynamic therapy in advanced tracheobronchial cancers. *Diagn Ther Endosc.* 1999;5(4):245-51.

[49] Kato H, Okunaka T, Tsuchida T, Shibuya H, Fujino S, Ogawa K. Analysis of the Cost-effectiveness of Photodynamic Therapy in Early Stage Lung Cancer. *Diagn Ther Endosc.* 1999;6(1):9-16.

[50] Okunaka T, Hiyoshi T, Furukawa K, Yamamoto H, Tsuchida T, Usuda J, Kumasaka H, Ishida J, Konaka C, Kato H. Lung cancers treated with photodynamic therapy and surgery. *Diagn Ther Endosc.* 1999;5(3):155-60.

[51] McCaughan JS. Photodynamic therapy for obstructive esophageal malignancies. *Diagn Ther Endosc.* 1999;5(3):167-74.

[52] Mimura S, Narahara H, Otani T, Okuda S. Progress of photodynamic therapy in gastric cancer. *Diagn Ther Endosc.* 1999;5(3):175-82.

[53] MacCormack MA. Photodynamic therapy in dermatology: an update on applications and outcomes. *Semin Cutan Med Surg.* 2008 Mar;27(1):52-62.

[54] Ostrow JD, Wennberg RP, Tiribelli C. Phototherapy for neonatal jaundice. *N Engl J Med.* 2008 Jun 5;358(23):2524

[55] Boo NY, Chew EL. A randomised control trial of clingfilm for prevention of hypothermia in term infants during phototherapy. *Singapore Med J.* 2006 Sep;47(9):757-62.

[56] Djokomuljanto S, Quah BS, Surini Y, Noraida R, Ismail NZ, Hansen TW, Van Rostenberghe H. Efficacy of phototherapy for neonatal jaundice is increased by the use of low-cost white reflecting curtains. *Arch Dis Child Fetal Neonatal Ed.* 2006 Nov;91(6):F439-42.

[57] Yaseen H, Khalaf M, Rashid N, Darwich M. Does prophylactic phototherapy prevent hyperbilirubinemia in neonates with ABO incompatibility and positive Coombs' test? *J Perinatol.* 2005 Sep;25(9):590-4.

[58] Bader D, Kugelman A, Blum DE, Riskin A, Tirosh E. Effect of phototherapy on cardiorespiratory activity during sleep in neonates with physiologic jaundice. *Isr Med Assoc J.* 2006 Jan;8(1):12-6.

[59] Murki S, Dutta S, Narang A, Sarkar U, Garewal G. A randomized, triple-blind, placebo-controlled trial of prophylactic oral phenobarbital to reduce the need for phototherapy in G6PD-deficient neonates. *J Perinatol.* 2005 May;25(5):325-30.

[60] Mohammadzadeh A, Bostani Z, Jafarnejad F, Mazloom R. Supine versus turning position on bilirubin level during phototherapy in healthy term jaundiced neonates. *Saudi Med J.* 2004 Dec;25(12):2051-2.

[61] Turan O, Ergenekon E, Koç E, Atalay Y, Unal S, Gücüyener K, Erbaş D, Seneş M. Impact of phototherapy on vasoactive mediators: NO and VEGF in the newborn. *J Perinat Med.* 2004;32(4):359-64.

Chapter X

GENE TRANSFER AND GENE THERAPY

INTRODUCTION TO GENOMICS

A. History of Genetics

At the starting point of this century genetics arose out of developmental history as the science of the reasonable understanding of development [1]. The concept of the difference between the possibility for a trait and the trait proper, between the genotype and the phenotype, was clear only during the first decade of the century [2]. After Spemann's epochal discovery, who already rewarded with the Nobel Prize in 1935, of the organizer and the beginning of the experimental analysis of developmental fields, little or no progress was derived until the last few years when a new emerging revolution appeared in developmental biology [1]. The classical point of view prevailed into the 1930s, and conceived the gene as an indivisible single item of genetic transmission, recombination, mutation, and function [3]. The discovery of intragenic recombination in the early 1940s and the setting of DNA as the physical basis of inheritance resulted in the neoclassical concept of the gene, which prevailed until the 1970s [3].

In the past, studying of the gene is not easy but very difficult. Genetic laboratory seems to be a complex and mysterious field. The discoveries of DNA technology, beginning in the early 1970s, have resulted in the second revolution in the concept of the gene in which none of the classical or neoclassical criteria for the definition of the gene hold extremely true [4]. These are several new findings concerning gene repetition and overlapping, movable genes, complex promoters, multiple polyadenylation sites, polyprotein genes, editing of the primary transcript, pseudogenes and gene nesting [4]. Introduction of Southern, Northern and dot blotting and DNA sequencing later in the 1970s considerably improved the diagnostic capabilities [5]. Nevertheless, it was the new finding of the polymerase chain reaction (PCR) in 1985 that resulted in an exponential blooming in molecular biology and the introduction of practicable nucleic acid tests in the routine laboratory [5]. Blooming of molecular biology leads to several simplified techniques for genetic studying. Finding amino acid sequence of a gene can be easily done by basic sequencing technique.

B. What is Genomics?

In a basic classical word, genomics is the study of genome. This is the first "omic" science appeared in bioinformatics. The availability of a complete microbial genome sequence in 1995 brought the first setting of a genomic era that has allowed medical scientists to change the paradigm and approach vaccine development starting from genomic data [6]. The whole-genome perspective is expected to give an instrumental contribution to drug and vaccine development, particularly to target those pathogenic agents for which the traditional approaches have failed so far [7]. Combining pathogen genome sequences with the host and vector genome sequences is promising to become a robust mean for the identification of host-pathogen interactions [8]. In additional, comparative sequencing of related species, especially of organisms used as model systems in the study of the pathogenic disorder, is starting to realize its potential in the identification of genes that are involved in evasion of the host immune response [8]. The root of genomics is genetics, which is a medical science with very long history. However, the start of genomics is appeared in the post-genome era. Completeness of genome project is noted to be the starting point of genomics. Bioinformatics has become an integral part of research and development in new advanced biomedical sciences. The field of bioinformatics is at the heart point of functional and genomics and advances will rely on the continuing evolution of tools to interpret data [9].

C. Gene Identification

It is quite common for molecular biologists to sequence genes or their fragments whose functions are primarily unknown. To identify gene from these findings are the focus. cDNAs is a useful basic application for gene identification. A cDNA library, containing clones for thousands of genes, can be set using mRNA from almost any tissue from any species. When a cDNA has been completely determined, it is referred to as an Expressed Sequence Tag (EST). Since different genes are expressed in different tissues, at different points in development, and under different environmental conditions, EST can assist to find out which genes, and which biochemical pathways, are significant in different cellular contexts. The technology of sequencing ESTs provides a relatively inexpensive alternative to whole genome sequencing and has become a proper resource for gene discovery. Identification of genes in a genomic DNA sequence can be presently done based on bioinformatics techniques. Prediction of protein-coding genes is the first start for gene identification. The next step is the computation prediction by software.

D. Concept for Gene Therapy

Gene therapy is an appication of gene knowledge on medical treatment. This is the new hope in medicine. This can be a big jump for medical treatment. Concept of gene therapy has been set for a few years. Gene therapy means usage of gene for treatment. Because gene is the basic unit that will further transform the data into the expression via proteome. Therefore, modification and manipulation of gene can be the clue for treatment of many gene-based disorder. This can be done at present. Based on the concept of gene therapy, the necessary steps include 1) gene identification, 2) gene selection, 3) gene transfer and 4) monitoring of result. Gene identification is the identification of problematic gene. This can be done by basic gene knowledge and bioinformatics technique as previously mentioned. Gene selection is the selection of appropriate gene aiming at function for treatment for each case. Gene tranfer is the transferring of desired selected gene into the pathogeneic gene part. The final step is monitoring of treatment result which is the basic requirement for all medical treatments.

MEDICAL ETHICS FOR GENE THERAPY

Table 1. Some important reports on medical ethics for gene therapy

authors	details
Ebbesen et al. [10]	Ebbesen et al. reported on ethical perspectives on RNA interference therapeutics [10]. Ebbesen et al. said that the ethical issues in RNA interference therapeutics not only included a risk-benefit analysis, but also considerations about respecting the autonomy of the patient and considerations about justice with regard to the inclusion criteria for participation in clinical trials and health care allocation [10].
Jin et al. [11]	Jin et al. discussed on ethics on gene therapy for liver disease [11].
Anderson [12]	Anderson discussed on ethical preparedness and performance of gene therapy study co-ordinators [12].
Kimmelman [13]	Kimmelman discussed on the ethics of human gene transfer [13]. Kimmelman said that the main question were when to initiate human testing, the acceptability of germline modification and whether the technique should be applied to the enhancement of traits [13].
Kahn [14]	Kahn discussed on informed consent for gene therapy [14].
Silber [15]	Silber discussed on informed consent for gene therapy [15].
Bruce [16]	Bruce discussed on moral and ethical issues in gene therapy [16].
Bleijs et al. [17]	Bleijs et al. discussed on gene therapy in the Netherland [17].

Because gene therapy is a new technology it is a focused area in medical ethics. Gene therapy is a big question because the induction of mutation can bring uncontrollable disaster if it has any defect. This is a good ethical dilemma scenario of the situation when science intersects with standard ethical principles. Similar to stem cell therapy, the appropriate solution must be a mid way position that would support the advancement of science for the benefit of human, while maintaining the ethics. This balance status would be a key success for sustainable science and society development for real application of gene therapy technology. Another important notification is that gene therapy can be the invasion to god in the context of religion. Can we modify the god's code? This is a very complicated issue. Some important reports on medical ethics for stem cell therapy will be listed in Table 1.

Gene Transfer

Gene transfer is an important step in gene therapy. This is the transferring of genetic content to new site. Guo et al. said that natural and synthetic enhancer-promoters could be used to drive gene transcription in a temporal, spatial or environmental signal-inducible manner in response to heat shock, hypoxia, radiation, chemotherapy, epigenetic agents or viral infection [18]. Guo et al. also noted that a regulatable gene-expression system could also be implemented to allow tightly regulated expression [18]. The vector is used for transferring. Vilaboa and Voellmy noted that the most commonly considered gene switches that are reviewed herein are based on small molecule-responsive transactivators derived from bacterial tetracycline repressor, insect or mammalian steroid receptors, or mammalian FKBP12/FRAP [19]. A wide variety of viral expression systems have been used and assessed for their ability to transfer genes into somatic cells [20]. In particular, retroviral and adenoviral mediated gene transfer was extensively studied [20]. Walther and Stein said that preclinical and clinical studies covering a wide range of genetic disorders were underway to solve basic issues dealing with gene transfer efficiencies, regulation of gene expression, and potential risks of the use of viral vectors [20]. Some important reports on gene transfer will be hereby presented in Table 2.

Gene Therapy

A. Arbovirus and Gene Therapy

In addition to gene transfer, several arboviruses can be used for novel gene therapy. Semliki Forest virus is the one that is frequently used for gene therapy. The CNS gene therapy by Semliki Forest virus is widely researched. Tuittila et al. noted that induction of proinflammatory cytokine mRNA in the CNS by SFV infection seemed to correlate with the rate of viral replication and was not importantly influenced by the virus envelope or nonstructural protein primary structure Semliki Forest virus [34]. They said that the outcomes had relevance for development of CNS gene therapy vectors as SFV4 and A774 display differences in CNS infection characteristics [34]. However, Graham et al. reported that the current SFV1 vector system was limited in its property for CNS gene therapy by neurotoxicity [35]. In addition to CNS gene therapy, the use of Semliki Forest virus in cancer gene therapy is widely mentioned in the literature. It was observed that that recombinant particles, naked RNA and plasmid DNA containing Semliki Forest virus replicons, could demonstrate a strong immune response against recombinantly expressed proteins, which had shown preventive action against tumor challenges [36]. Intratumoural injection of Semliki Forest virus particles had led to tumor regression [36]. Colmenero et al. reported that immunotherapy with recombinant Semliki Forest virus -replicons expressing the P815A tumor antigen or interleukin-12 (IL-12) could lead to tumor regression [37]. Murphy et al. reported an inhibition of human lung cancer cell growth by apoptosis induction using Semliki Forest virus recombinant particles [38]. In their study [38], direct injection of rSFV into H358a tumors subcutaneously implanted as xenografts in nu/nu mice inhibited tumor growth, and in some studied subjects caused absolute regression [38]. It is concluded that tumor growth suppression induced by rSFV was owing to apoptosis induction and that the vector has an inherent cell death-promoting and antitumor activity [38]. Asselin-Paturel et al. reported that transfer of the murine interleukin-12 gene in vivo by a Semliki Forest virus vector could lead to B16 tumor regression through inhibition of tumor blood vessel formation monitored by Doppler ultrasonography [39]. In 2007, Lyons et al. reported a similar observation in their study that active immunization with rSFV particles coding for VEGFR-2 could break immunological tolerance and could potentially be applied as part of a new treatment for cancer [40]. They reported that co-immunization of mice with rSFV particles encoding vascular endothelial growth factor receptor-2 (VEGFR-2) and IL-12 completely abrogated both the antibody result and the antitumor activity [40]. Prevention of angiogenesis by a Semliki Forest virus vector expressing VEGFR-2 reduces tumour growth and metastasis in mice is proposed [41]. This result is similar to another report by Chikkanna-Gowda et al. in 2005 [41]. Indeed, the induction of a therapeutic antitumor immunological response by intratumoral injection of genetically engineered Semliki Forest virus to cause IL-12 was published by Yamanaka et al. since 2000 [42].

Sindbis virus is also proposed for its effectiveness in gene therapy for several cancers [43]. Hay noted that a recent report demonstrates that the Sindbis virus had significant properties in three challenging areas of gene therapy - specificity, efficacy and delivery, suggesting that Sindbis had the feasibility to become a good gene therapy vector for cancer therapy [43]. Cancer immunotherapy by Sindbis virus is the new way in the cancer treatment. Cheng et al. recently used the replication-defective vaccine vector Sindbis virus replicon particles from a modern packaging cell line (PCL) to contruct Sindbis virus replicon particles encoding calreticulin (CRT) linked to a model tumor antigen, HPV16 E7 protein [43]. Cheng et al. created a recombinant Sindbis virus -based replicon particle encoding VP22 linked to a model tumor antigen, human papillomavirus type 16 (HPV-16) E7, making use of a stable SIN PCL [44]. According to this study, Sindbis virus replicon particles encoding calreticulin linked to a tumor antigen caused long-term tumor-specific immunity [44]. Cheng et al. concluded that the CRT strategy used in the context of SIN replicon particles facilitated the generation of a significantly effective vaccine for cancer prophylaxis and immunotherapy [44]. Cheng et al. also indicated that the VP22, a herpes simplex virus type 1 (HSV-1) tegument protein, strategy applied in the context of Sindbis virus replicon particles might enhance the generation of a highly effective vaccine for widespread immunization [45]. Zhnag et al. reasoned that Sindbis-virus-based vectors might be good for gibbon ape leukemia virus envelope glycoprotein (GALV.fus) gene transfer because high-titer stocks can easily be caused in hamster cells and Sindbis virus efficiently infects human tumor cells through the high-affinity 67 kDa laminin receptor [46]. They reported that Sindbis vectors expressing GALV.fus could be packaged into contagious viral particles to high titer, exhibited potent bystander cytopathic activity and were active against U87 glioma xenografts [28]. They concluded that Sindbis-virus-based replicons was efficient vector systems for delivery and expression of fusogenic membrane glycoproteins [46]. In 1998, Swai and Meruelo explored the possibility of designing a Sindbis virus vector that could attack human choriocarcinoma cells via ligand-receptor interaction [47]. In this study, the hCG-envelope chimeric virus vector had minimal infectivities against BHK cells and human cancer cells which did not pose LH/CG receptors on their surface [47]. Swai and Meruelo proposed that the chimeric Sindbis virus vector may bring a novel approach for gene therapy of gestational trophoblast disease and placental dysfunction [47]. Bergman attempted to construct a virus that targeted specifically to breast cancer cells [48]. In their attempt, nonreplicating and replicating pseudotype Vesicular stomatitis virus (VSV) were constructed whose only surface glycoprotein (gp) was a Sindbis gp, called Sindbis-ZZ, modified to severely decrease its native binding function and to contain the Fc-binding domain of *Staphylococcus aureus* protein A [48]. Bergman et al. reported that vesicular stomatitis virus expressing a chimeric Sindbis glycoprotein containing an Fc antibody binding domain could attack to Her2/neu overexpressing breast cancer cells [48]. This work demonstrates the ability to easily create, directly from plasmid components, an oncolytic replicating VSV with a restricted host cell range [48]. Morizono et al. reported successful targeting in a living animal through intravenous injection of a lentiviral vector pseudotyped with a adapted chimeric Sindbis virus envelope (termed m168) [49]. They found that m168 pseudotypes had high titer and high targeting specificity and, unlike other retroviral pseudotypes, had low nonspecific infectivity in hepatic and spleen [49]. According to this study, human P-glycoprotein was ectopically demonstrated on the surface of melanoma cells and attacked by the m168 pseudotyped lentiviral vector conjugated with antibody specific for P-glycoprotein. m168 pseudotypes successfully attacked metastatic melanoma cells growing in the lung after systemic administration by tail vein injection [50].

B. Adenovirus and Gene Therapy

In addition to gene transfer, adenovirus can be used for novel gene therapy [51]. Basically, adenovirus type 5 E1A gene as a potential therapeutic gene in breast and ovarian cancer since 1995 by using cationic liposome as gene delivery system [51-58]. Therapeutic transfer of DNA encoding adenoviral E1A is the best scenario [52].

Deissler and Opalka said that therapeutic applications of E1A were covered by a series of patents which include the description of small variants that could be used for tumor suppression and E1A gene transfer in combination with conventional chemotherapy [52]. Liao et al. also reported on enhanced paclitaxel cytotoxicity and prolonged animal survival rate by a nonviral-mediated systemic delivery of E1A gene in orthotopic xenograft human breast cancer [53]. In addition, Zang et al. reported that adenovirus-type 5 E1a gene could efficaciously prevent HER-2/neu-overexpressing ovarian cancer, and this promising procedure could greatly benefit ovarian cancer patients with high expression of HER-2/neu [54]. Yu et al. also proposed that liposome-mediated in vivo E1A gene transfer suppressed dissemination of ovarian cancer cells that overexpress HER-2/neu [55]. However, Xing et al. reported on safety study and characterization of E1A-liposome complex gene-delivery protocol in an ovarian cancer model [56]. Xing et al. reported that resistance of the E1A DNA extracted from tissues to the digestion of Dpnl restriction enzyme, which could cleave the methylated E1A plasmid DNA generated by methylation-competent bacteria, implied possible integration of E1A DNA into the chromosome of the lungs and kidneys during therapy and brought a question on safety of this protocol [56].

Sang et al. said that E1A should be utilized to make continuous contributions not only to a better understanding of the molecular mechanisms underlying the regulation of transcription, cell division, apoptosis and tumorigenesis but also to modern therapeutics such as gene therapy [57].

Table 2. Some important reports on gene transfer in gene therapy

authors	details
Goins et al. [21]	Goins et al. reported on construction and production of recombinant herpes simplex virus vectors [21].
Lee and Mohapatra [22]	Lee and Mohapatra reported on chitosan nanoparticle-mediated gene transfer [22].
Palmer and Ng [23]	Palmer and Ng reported on methods for the production of first generation adenoviral vectors [23]. Palmer and Ng noted that adenoviruses could efficiently infect a wide variety of quiescent and proliferating cell types from various species to direct high level viral gene expression and their 36 kb double-stranded DNA genome could be modified with relative ease by classical molecular biology techniques, and could be readily propagated and purified to yield high titer preparations of very stable virus [23].
Souied et al. [24]	Souied et al. reported on non-invasive gene transfer by iontophoresis for therapy of an inherited retinal degeneration [24].
Kanemura et al. [25]	Kanemura et al. reported on hepatocyte growth factor gene transfer with naked plasmid DNA ameliorates dimethylnitrosamine-induced liver fibrosis in rats [25].
Bowman et al. [26]	Bowman et al. reported on gene transfer to hemophilia A mice via oral delivery of FVIII-chitosan nanoparticles [26].
Müller et al. [27]	Müller et al. reported on augmentation of AAV-mediated cardiac gene transfer after systemic administration in adult rats [27].
Jin et al. [28]	Jin et al. reported on adenovirus-mediated gene transfer of interleukin-23 shows prophylactic but not therapeutic antitumor effects [28].
Feshe [29]	Feshe reported on Clinical application of a retroviral gene transfer protocol based on centrifugation-mediated vector preloading [29].
Moon et al. [30]	Moon et al. reported on efficient bone marrow transduction by gene transfer with allogeneic umbilical cord blood serum and plasma: an implication for clinical trials [30].
Sebestyén et al. [31]	Sebestyén et al. found that human TCR that incorporated CD3zeta could induce highly preferred pairing between TCRalpha and beta chains following gene transfer [31].
Santoni de Sio et al. [32]	Santoni de Sio et al. found that the proteasome limited lentiviral gene transfer in all stem cell types tested, including embryonic, mesenchymal and neural, both of human and mouse origin [32].
Verhoeyen et al. [33]	Verhoeyen et al. described the production of a new early acting cytokine displaying vectors and the methodology to confirm the capacity of these vectors to promote selective transduction of hematopoietic stem cells [33].

C. *Escherichia Coli* and Gene Therapy

Escherichia coli is also applied for gene therapy. It is the most widely used non viral vector [58]. Therapeutic benefits of *E.coli* –based gene modification have been observed in vaccination against infectious diseases, immunotherapy against cancer, and topical delivery of immunomodulatory cytokines in inflammatory bowel disease [59]. *E.coli* purine nucleoside phosphorylase (PNP) which catalyzes the cleavage of 9-(2-deoxy-beta-D-ribofuranosyl)-6-methylpurine (MeP-dR) is widely applied for gene therapy [60]. The development of *E. coli* PNP anticancer gene therapy was the novel in this area [60]. Recently, Cai et al. reported on experimental studies on PNP suicide gene therapy of hepatoma [61]. Cai et al. concluded that high-level bystander effects of this system resulted in significant anti-tumor responses to hepatoma gene therapy, especially in vivo [61]. Hughes et al. also reported on Bystander killing of melanoma cells using this system [62].

REFERENCES

[1] Opitz JM. Developmental disorders of man. Part 2. *Monatsschr Kinderheilkd.* 1992 May;140(5):264-72.

[2] Falk R. The gene in search of an identity. *Hum Genet.* 1984;68(3):195-204.

[3] Portin P. The concept of the gene: short history and present status. *Q Rev Biol.* 1993 Jun;68(2):173-223.

[4] Portin P. Historical development of the concept of the gene. *J Med Philos.* 2002 Jun;27(3):257-86.

[5] Csako G. Present and future of rapid and/or high-throughput methods for nucleic acid testing. *Clin Chim Acta.* 2006 Jan;363(1-2):6-31.

[6] Serruto D, Rappuoli R. Post-genomic vaccine development. *FEBS Lett.* 2006, 580: 2985-92.

[7] Scarselli M, Giuliani MM, Adu-Bobie J, Pizza M, Rappuoli R. The impact of genomics on vaccine design. *Trends Biotechnol.* 2005, 23: 84-91.

[8] Capecchi B, Serruto D, Adu-Bobie J, Rappuoli R, Pizza M. The genome revolution in vaccine research. *Curr Issues Mol Biol.* 2004, 6: 17-27.

[9] Mundy C. The human genome project: a historical perspective. *Pharmacogenomics.* 2001 Feb;2(1):37-49.

[10] Ebbesen M, Jensen TG, Andersen S, Pedersen FS. Ethical perspectives on RNA interference therapeutics. *Int J Med Sci.* 2008 Jun 25;5(3):159-68.

[11] Jin X, Yang YD, Li YM. Gene therapy: regulations, ethics and its practicalities in liver disease. *World J Gastroenterol.* 2008 Apr 21;14(15):2303-7.

[12] Anderson G. Ethical preparedness and performance of gene therapy study co-ordinators. *Nurs Ethics.* 2008 Mar;15(2):208-21.

[13] Kimmelman J. The ethics of human gene transfer. *Nat Rev Genet.* 2008 Mar;9(3):239-44.

[14] Kahn J. Informed consent in human gene transfer clinical trials. *Hum Gene Ther.* 2008 Jan;19(1):7-8.

[15] Silber TJ. Human gene therapy, consent, and the realities of clinical research: is it time for a research subject advocate? *Hum Gene Ther.* 2008 Jan;19(1):11-4.

[16] Bruce DM. Moral and ethical issues in gene therapy. *Hum Reprod Genet Ethics.* 2006;12(1):16-23.

[17] Bleijs DA, Haenen IT, Bergmans JE. Gene therapy legislation in The Netherlands. *J Gene Med.* 2007 Oct;9(10):904-9.

[18] Guo ZS, Li Q, Bartlett DL, Yang JY, Fang B. Gene transfer: the challenge of regulated gene expression. *Trends Mol Med.* 2008 Aug 7. [Epub ahead of print]

[19] Vilaboa N, Voellmy R. Regulatable gene expression systems for gene therapy. *Curr Gene Ther.* 2006 Aug;6(4):421-38.

[20] Walther W, Stein U. Cell type specific and inducible promoters for vectors in gene therapy as an approach for cell targeting. *J Mol Med.* 1996 Jul;74(7):379-92.

[21] Goins WF, Krisky DM, Wechuck JB, Huang S, Glorioso JC. Construction and production of recombinant herpes simplex virus vectors. *Methods Mol Biol.* 2008;433:97-113.

[22] Lee D, Mohapatra SS. Chitosan nanoparticle-mediated gene transfer. *Methods Mol Biol.* 2008;433:127-40.

[23] Palmer DJ, Ng P. Methods for the production of first generation adenoviral vectors. *Methods Mol Biol.* 2008;433:55-78.

[24] Souied EH, Reid SN, Piri NI, Lerner LE, Nusinowitz S, Farber DB. Non-invasive gene transfer by iontophoresis for therapy of an inherited retinal degeneration. *Exp Eye Res.* 2008 Apr 29. [Epub ahead of print]

[25] Kanemura H, Iimuro Y, Takeuchi M, Ueki T, Hirano T, Horiguchi K, Asano Y, Fujimoto J. Hepatocyte growth factor gene transfer with naked plasmid DNA ameliorates dimethylnitrosamine-induced liver fibrosis in rats. *Hepatol Res.* 2008 Jul 9. [Epub ahead of print]

[26] Bowman K, Sarkar R, Raut S, Leong KW. Gene transfer to hemophilia A mice via oral delivery of FVIII-chitosan nanoparticles. *J Control Release.* 2008 Jun 27. [Epub ahead of print]

[27] Müller OJ, Schinkel S, Kleinschmidt JA, Katus HA, Bekeredjian R. Augmentation of AAV-mediated cardiac gene transfer after systemic administration in adult rats. *Gene Ther.* 2008 Jul 10. [Epub ahead of print]

[28] Jin HT, Youn JI, Choi SY, Seo SH, Park SH, Song MY, Yang SH, Sung YC. Adenovirus-mediated gene transfer of interleukin-23 shows prophylactic but not therapeutic antitumor effects. *Cancer Gene Ther.* 2008 Jul 4. [Epub ahead of print]

[29] Fehse B. Clinical application of a retroviral gene transfer protocol based on centrifugation-mediated vector preloading. *Hum Gene Ther.* 2008 Jun;19(6):655-6.

[30] Moon N, Yang SJ, Park BB, Chung YS, Lee JW, Oh IH. Efficient bone marrow transduction by gene transfer with allogeneic umbilical cord blood serum and plasma: an implication for clinical trials. *Hum Gene Ther.* 2008 Jul;19(7):744-52.

[31] Sebestyén Z, Schooten E, Sals T, Zaldivar I, San José E, Alarcón B, Bobisse S, Rosato A, Szöllosi J, Gratama JW, Willemsen RA, Debets Human TCR that incorporate CD3zeta induce highly preferred pairing between TCRalpha and beta chains following gene transfer. *J Immunol.* 2008 Jun 1;180(11):7736-46.

[32] Santoni de Sio FR, Gritti A, Cascio P, Neri M, Sampaolesi M, Galli C, Luban J, Naldini L. Lentiviral Vector Gene Transfer is Limited by the Proteasome at Post-Entry Steps in Various Types of Stem Cells. *Stem Cells*. 2008 May 15. [Epub ahead of print]

[33] Verhoeyen E, Nègre D, Cosset FL. Production of lentiviruses displaying "early-acting" cytokines for selective gene transfer into hematopoietic stem cells. *Methods Mol Biol*. 2008;434:99-112.

[34] Schvartzman JB, Parras LM, Krimer DB. Replication and segregation of eukaryotic chromosomal DNA. *Revis Biol Celular*. 1986;10:1-130.

[35] Tuittila M, Nygardas P, Hinkkanen A. mRNA expression of proinflammatory cytokines in mouse CNS correlates with replication rate of semliki forest virus but not with the strain of viral proteins. *Viral. Immunol. 17*, 287-97 (2004)

[36] Graham A, Walker R, Baird P, Hahn CN, Fazakerley JK. CNS gene therapy applications of the Semliki Forest virus 1 vector are limited by neurotoxicity. *Mol. Ther. 13*, 631-5 (2006)

[37] Colmenero P, Chen M, Castanos-Velez E, Liljestrom P, Jondal M. Immunotherapy with recombinant SFV-replicons expressing the P815A tumor antigen or IL-12 induces tumor regression. *Int. J. Cancer. 98*, 554-60 (2002)

[38] Murphy AM, Morris-Downes MM, Sheahan BJ, Atkins GJ. Inhibition of human lung carcinoma cell growth by apoptosis induction using Semliki Forest virus recombinant particles. *Gene. Ther. 7*, 1477-82 (2000)

[39] Asselin-Paturel C, Lassau N, Guinebretiere JM, Zhang J, Gay F, Bex F, Hallez S, Leclere J, Peronneau P, Mami-Chouaib F, Chouaib S. Transfer of the murine interleukin-12 gene in vivo by a Semliki Forest virus vector induces B16 tumor regression through inhibition of tumor blood vessel formation monitored by Doppler ultrasonography. *Gene. Ther. 6*, 606-15 (1999)

[40] Lyons JA, Sheahan BJ, Galbraith SE, Mehra R, Atkins GJ, Fleeton MN. Inhibition of angiogenesis by a Semliki Forest virus vector expressing VEGFR-2 reduces tumour growth and metastasis in mice. *Gene. Ther. 14*, 503-13 (2007)

[41] Chikkanna-Gowda CP, Sheahan BJ, Fleeton MN, Atkins GJ. Regression of mouse tumours and inhibition of metastases following administration of a Semliki Forest virus vector with enhanced expression of IL-12. *Gene. Ther. 12*, 1253-63 (2005)

[42] Yamanaka R, Zullo SA, Tanaka R, Ramsey J, Blaese M, Xanthopoulos KG. Induction of a therapeutic antitumor immunological response by intratumoral injection of genetically engineered Semliki Forest virus to produce interleukin-12. Neurosurg. Focus. 9, e7 (2000)

[43] Hay JG. Sindbis virus--an effective targeted cancer therapeutic. *Trends. Biotechnol. 22*, 501-3 (2004)

[44] Cheng WF, Lee CN, Su YN, Chai CY, Chang MC, Polo JM, Hung CF, Wu TC, Hsieh CY, Chen CA. Sindbis virus replicon particles encoding calreticulin linked to a tumor antigen generate long-term tumor-specific immunity. *Cancer. Gene. Ther. 13*, 873-85 (2006)

[45] Cheng WF, Hung CF, Hsu KF, Chai CY, He L, Polo JM, Slater LA, Ling M, Wu TC. Cancer immunotherapy using Sindbis virus replicon particles encoding a VP22-antigen fusion. *Hum Gene Ther*. 2002; 13: 553-68.

[46] Zhang J, Frolov I, Russell SJ. Gene therapy for malignant glioma using Sindbis vectors expressing a fusogenic membrane glycoprotein. *J Gene Med*. 2004; 6: 1082-91.

[47] Sawai K, Meruelo D. Cell-specific transfection of choriocarcinoma cells by using Sindbis virus hCG expressing chimeric vector. *Biochem. Biophys. Res. Commun*. 1998; 248: 315-23.

[48] Bergman I, Whitaker-Dowling P, Gao Y, Griffin JA, Watkins SC. Vesicular stomatitis virus expressing a chimeric Sindbis glycoprotein containing an Fc antibody binding domain targets to Her2/neu overexpressing breast cancer cells. *Virology*. 2003; 316: 337-47.

[49] Morizono K, Xie Y, Ringpis GE, Johnson M, Nassanian H, Lee B, Wu L, Chen IS. Lentiviral vector retargeting to P-glycoprotein on metastatic melanoma through intravenous injection. *Nat Med*. 2005; 11: 346-52.

[50] Polo JM, Gardner JP, Ji Y, Belli BA, Driver DA, Sherrill S, Perri S, Liu MA, Dubensky TW Jr. Alphavirus DNA and particle replicons for vaccines and gene therapy. *Dev Biol (Basel)*. 2000;104:181-5.

[51] Segura MM, Alba R, Bosch A, Chillón M. Advances in helper-dependent adenoviral vector research. *Curr Gene Ther*. 2008 Aug;8(4):222-35.

[52] Deissler H, Opalka B. Therapeutic transfer of DNA encoding adenoviral E1A. *Recent Patents Anticancer Drug Discov*. 2007 Jan;2(1):1-10.

[53] Liao Y, Zou YY, Xia WY, Hung MC. Enhanced paclitaxel cytotoxicity and prolonged animal survival rate by a nonviral-mediated systemic delivery of E1A gene in orthotopic xenograft human breast cancer. *Cancer Gene Ther*. 2004 Sep;11(9):594-602.

[54] Zang RY, Shi DR, Lu HJ, Cai SM, Lu DR, Zhang YJ, Qin HL. Adenovirus 5 E1a-mediated gene therapy for human ovarian cancer cells in vitro and in vivo. *Int J Gynecol Cancer*. 2001 Jan-Feb;11(1):18-23.

[55] Yu D, Matin A, Xia W, Sorgi F, Huang L, Hung MC. Liposome-mediated in vivo E1A gene transfer suppressed dissemination of ovarian cancer cells that overexpress HER-2/neu. *Oncogene*. 1995 Oct 5;11(7):1383-8.

[56] Xing X, Zhang S, Chang JY, Tucker SD, Chen H, Huang L, Hung MC. Safety study and characterization of E1A-liposome complex gene-delivery protocol in an ovarian cancer model. *Gene Ther*. 1998 Nov;5(11):1538-44.

[57] Sang N, Caro J, Giordano A. Adenoviral E1A: everlasting tool, versatile applications, continuous contributions and new hypotheses. *Front Biosci*. 2002 Feb 1;7:d407-13.

[58] Ueno NT, Yu D, Hung MC. E1A: tumor suppressor or oncogene? Preclinical and clinical investigations of E1A gene therapy. *Breast Cancer*. 2001;8(4):285-93.

[59] Voss C. Production of plasmid DNA for pharmaceutical use. *Biotechnol Annu Rev*. 2007;13:201-22.

[60] Zhang Y, Parker WB, Sorscher EJ, Ealick SE. PNP anticancer gene therapy. *Curr Top Med Chem*. 2005;5(13):1259-74.

[61] Cai X, Zhou J, Lin J, Sun X, Xue X, Li C. Experimental studies on PNP suicide gene therapy of hepatoma. *J Huazhong Univ Sci Technolog Med Sci.* 2005;25(2):178-81.

[62] Hughes BW, Wells AH, Bebok Z, Gadi VK, Garver RI Jr, Parker WB, Sorscher EJ. Bystander killing of melanoma cells using the human tyrosinase promoter to express the Escherichia coli purine nucleoside phosphorylase gene. *Cancer Res.* 1995 Aug 1;55(15):3339-45.

Chapter XI

IMMUNOTHERAPY

WHAT IS IMMUNITY? [1-8]

The word immunity is a basic medical word describing a specific system of human beings. Immunity is a specific system dealing with the defensive mechanism. Everyday, human body has to expose to several alien foreign bodies and some of these alien foreign bodies are harmful and needs proper management. Immunity plays important roles for this overall process. Considering defensive mechanism of human beings, there are 2 main parts immunity and non-immunity portions. Non-immunity portion is a non specific process and usually firstly act to any alien foreign bodies. Examples of non specific process are mucous barrier and several reflexes. Considering immunity, it is a specific process. The hallmarks of immunity consists of memory and specificity, therefore, the first exposure cannot generate immunity. The immunity process can be divided into two main parts: humoral mediated immunity and cellular mediated immunity. Humoral medicated immunity makes use of humoral substance, antibody for action. Whereas cellular mediated immunity makes use of cells, blood cells, for action. Of several cells in blood stream, lymphocyte, T cell, B cell and nonTnonB cell, are mentioned for cellular mediated immunity. These main kinds of lymphocytes take important role in cellular immune process. T cell takes role for generation of cytokine whereas B cell takes roles in antibody generation process.

As mentioned, immunity plays main roles in defensive mechanism. When a foreign body enters into human body and pass non specific immune defensive mechanism process, it will be further reacted by immunity. Destruction of foreign body can be seen via antibody system with help of compliment or via cell mediated immunity process with help of cytokine. With complete full function of immunity, pathogens or foreign bodies can be successfully destroyed. However, in some cases, those aliens can conquer immune system process and this will result in pathological conditions or diseases. Good examples are infections. With complete perfect immunity, human will be helpful. However, extremely high immunity process or hypersensitivity can be problematic. On the other hand, extremely low immunity process of immunity or immunodeficiency can also be problematic.

How can Immunity be Applied for Treatment?

As previously mentioned, immunity is useful for prevention, via destroying of foreign body that enters or invades into the human body before it can generate further problems. However, the present concept transform to the usage of immunity for medical treatment [9]. Schulte-Wissermann and Gardilcic wrote that this modification of immunity process would be helpful [9]. The immunotherapy is a new highlight in immunology. There are many forms of immune-related treatments. Important kinds will be hereby presented and briefly detailed.

A. Immunomodulation Therapy

Immunomodulation therapy is a new way of treatment making use of modification of immunity system to help curative process of some diseases. This is widely used for several treatments. More details can be further followed in the next part of this chapter.

B. Antibody Treatment

Antibody treatment is any treatment making use of administration of immunoglobulin or antibody. This is famous for a long time. Direct passive immunization is the good example. The most well-known situations are tetanus antitoxin injection and rabies immunoglobulin for preventive and therapeutic purposes. More details can be also further followed in the next part of this chapter.

C. Therapeutic Vaccination

Indeed vaccine is used for prevention and described as an active immunization. However, the present role of vaccine changes to more usefulness in curative treatment process. Therapeutic vaccination is the term used for this mentioned purpose. This specific kind of immunotherapy will be further discussed in another chapter in this book.

D. Cytokine Treatment

Cytokine treatment or cytokine therapy is another mode of immune – related treatment. Indeed, cytokine is a product in cellular process of cell-mediated immunity process. Cytokine treatment is used for medical treatment of many diseases especially for many viral infections. This is comparable to antibody treatment which makes usefulness of humoral immunity for treatment. The details of cytokine therapy will be summarized and presented in the following part in this chapter.

E. Immunogene Therapy [10]

Immunogene therapy is the newest modification of immunotherapy. This is the combination of the two concepts, immunotherapy and gene therapy. For more details on gene therapy, the readers can be read in another chapter in this book.

IMMUNOMODULATION THERAPY

Immunomodulation therapy can be performed with help of immunomodulator. There are several kinds of immunomodulators that are available for medical usage at present [11-13]. The author hereby will summarize on details of some important well-known immunomodulators.

A. Imiquimod [14]

Imiquimod is a new famous immunomodulative drug. Imiquimod is a new product recently introduced to physicians. Imiquimod, an imidazoquinoline amine, is a new immune response modifier agent recently approved for the local application in treatment of treatment of external genital and perianal warts [15-24]. Compared with the other routine therapeutic options for genital and perianal warts, imiquimod is less complicated to use and can be self-administrated by affected patients. Imiquimod poses no direct antiviral or antiproliferative activity when tested in a number of cell culture systems. Its activity for anti-herpes virus activity was accepted. One of the first analogs in the series, S -25059 was tested in the early 1980's and due to its slight toxicity, caused some reduction of pathology from herpes infection in cell cultures [15-17]. The dosage form of imiquimod is cream, generally known as ALDARA.(5) The chemical name of imiquimod is 1-(2-methylproply)-1 H-imidazol [4,5-c] quinolin - 4 – amine and its primary molecular formula is C14H16N4 [14]. Different from other immunomodulators, imiquimod is unique in that it activates immune function [25-38]. The exact mechanism of imiquimod's antiviral activity is not well described; however, its effects are likely to be related to its immunomodulating properties. Although *in vitro* studies have shown that imiquimod has no direct antiviral effects, the drug does exhibit antiviral and antitumor properties *in vivo* through induction of cytokines in human peripheral blood monocytes and increased cell-mediated cytolytic antiviral activity [25-38]. Imiquimod, and its. Much of the biologic activity of imiquimod compounds can be attributed to stimulate the innate immune response through the induction of cytokines and the cellular side of acquired immunity, covering interferon-alpha (IFN-alpha), interferon-gamma (IFN-gamma), tumor necrosis factoralpha, interleukins-1, -6, -8, -12 and others [14]. According to the animal experimental study, the concentrations of interferon and tumor necrosis factor were higher at the site of drug application than in skin from the cutaneous area from untreated animals [14]. Interferon-alpha mRNA levels were also increased in the cutaneous are of animal after topical application of imiquimod [14]. Imiquimod could also elevate interleukin-8 concentrations in human keratinocyte and fibroblast cultures [31,37]. But it did not lead to the transcriptional expression of inflammatory cytokines in human first trimester placental trophoblasts [26]. Therefore, stimulation of production of cytokines by imiquimod in the skin after local applications of the drug, may play a main function in its activity in genital wart patients [25-38].

Imiquimod, as first-line therapy, is the most cost-effective intervention comparing to other first-line or second-line alternative therapies. Therefore, consideration to use imiquimod cream as the first regimen for anogenital warts therapy is set, owing to the cost effectiveness [14]. The main clinical indication of imiquimod cream is for external genital, perianal warts and *condyloma accuminata* [14]. It is widely applied to treat the warts on surface of the penis or vulva and around the anus. No absolute contraindication is mentioned in the literature. But there is also no specific information from clinical trials for treatment of viral infections at other sites. Therefore, it is presently not recommended for usage for vaginal, cervix, rectal and anal infection in clinic [14]. The dermatological side effect at the lesion is the most common reported side effect of imiquimod [39-40]. Redness, ulceration, indurations, excoriation, flaking and edema can be observed. However, most of these skin reactions are usually mild to moderate [14]. Local erythema wand itching is the most common adverse reaction [39-40], but the main part of patients have no side effect or only mild local inflammatory reactions. Severe skin reaction can be observed in the case of imiquimod overdose [14].

Because imiquimod is a cytokine inducer, it can be successfully applied in the treatment of genital warts, a common sexual transmitted disease as previously mentioned. Several clinical trials have shown topical imiquimod to be effective and safe for the treatment of anogenital warts [41-46]. In addition, in clinical settings, patients responded well and wart recurrence rates appear to be lower than those reported for other classical therapies of genital warts.(29 - 34) The respond rate ranges from 75 to 100 % [41-46]. From analysis of the levels of expression of genes of the JAK/STAT signaling pathway and their inhibitors as well as IRFs in pretreatment biopsy collected specimens by reverse transcription-PCR, it is demonstrated that mRNA levels of signal transducer and activator of transcription 1 (STAT1) and IRF1 were higher in complete responders than in incomplete ones. Incomplete ones expressed larger amounts mRNA of STAT3, IRF2, and protein inhibitor of activated STAT1 (PIAS1) mRNAs compared to complete ones before imiquimod application. Therefore high-level expression of STAT1 and IRF1 is useful for a better response [25-38]. Treatment with imiquimod effectively elevates the mRNA level for interferon (IFN)-alpha, IFN-gamma and 2',5' oligoadenylate synthetase (2',5'- AS) as well as a tendency towards the elevation of tumor necrosis factor (TNF)-alpha and interleukin-12 p40 [14]. Notable increases in mRNA for CD4 and a trend toward increases in CD8 are also observed in imiquimod-treated cases [14]. Imiquimod administration is also related to a significant decrease in viral load as detectd by HPV DNA and L1 mRNA [14]. The effects on HPV markers are believed to become accompanied by an apparent reduction in mRNA expression for markers of cell proliferation and an increase in mRNA levels for biomarkers of keratinocyte differentiation and tumor suppressors [14]. From, randomized, double-blind, placebocontrolled studies, tropical imiquimod cream is effective and safe a self-administered therapy for external anogenital warts when used 3 times a week overnight for up to 4 months [14]. Furthermore, patients who received tropical imiquimod cream has more eradication of all treated baseline warts than other routine means [14]. Comparing to other currently available means for clearance of visible genital warts lesions, the failure rate, recurrence rate, and sideeffects of these treatments are usually low [41-46]. Imiquimod can be applied as patient self-directed regimen [14]. However, significant concerns in the use of this preparation included: firstly, patient education specifically for those who had previously received ablative therapy; secondly, the length of time that therapy would be continued prior to the patient was deemed to be a non-responder to this cream [14]. Good patient compliance should also be planned [14].

B. Levamisole

Levamisole, L-1-2, 3, 5, 6--tetrahydro-6- phenylimidazo (2, 1-b)-thiazol monohydrochloride, is another widely used immunomodulative drug. This is mentioned in many literatures for a long time. Levamisole is first introduced as a broad spectrum anthelmintic, an immunotherapeutic agent with anti-anergic properties, and is the first member of a potential new class of immunologically active, probably thymomimetic compounds [47]. Senn et al. said that levamisole increased colony formation, and altered colony-stimulating activity types detected in leucocyte-conditioned medium, makes this drug a promising candidate for treatment of selected leukaemic states and in preleukaemia [48]. Amery and Gough said that the main application of levamisol for immunotherapy was for immune deficiencies or as immune dysregulation syndromes such as rheumatoid arthritis and cancer [49]. Levamisole can play as an antianergic chemotherapeutic agent as it restores cell-mediated immunity in immunodepressed patients and extends the remission period [50]. It can expand the number of long-term survivors when used as an adjunct to cytoreductive therapy in several animal cancer experiment [50]. Levamisole can be absorbed from the gastrointestinal tract and from injection site and is extensively distributed in all tissues [50]. Levamisole also stimulates phagocytosis by polymorphonuclear cells or macrophages when added to the mentioned cells or given to donor animals and human beings [50-52]. Renoux said that immunomodulators given by modifying the functions of the host cells involved in defences against invaders, and the effectiveness of an immunotherapeutic drug relied on characteristics of the individual host, therefore, therapy with this drug should be individualized [53].

ANTIBODY TREATMENT

Antibody treatment makes use of administration of immunoglobulin or antibody for curative purpose. This is famous for a long time for many diseases. Good examples are tetanus, rabies and Kawasaki disease. Important interesting reports on antibody treatment will be given as idea to the readers in Table 2.

Table 1. Important reports on levamisole as immunomodulator

Authors	Details
Levy [54]	Levy reported on levamisole and cellular immunity in rheumatoid arthritis [54]. Reduced B cell function, immunoglobulin and autoantibody levels could be observed with levamisole treatment [54].
Taki and Schwartz [55]	Taki and Schwartz reported levamisole as an immunopotentiator for T cell deficiency [55].
Rosenthal et al. [56]	Rosenthal et al. reported on the effect of levamisole on peripheral blood lymphocyte subpopulations in patients with rheumatoid arthritis and ankylosing spondylitis [56].
Runge and Rynes [57]	Runge and Rynes discussed on balancing effectiveness and toxicity of levamisole in the treatment of rheumatoid arthritis [57]. Runge and Rynes said that because effective doses were poorly tolerated, and tolerable lower doses were relatively ineffective, levamisole was not recommended as standard treatment of rheumatoid arthritis [57].
Giulling et al. [58]	Giulling et al. reported on prediction of the effectiveness of levamisole immunotherapy by the sensitivity of blood lymphocytes to the drug [58].
Lvey [59]	Levy reported on correlations of clinical and laboratory effects of treatment with levamisole in autoimmune disease [59]. Levy concluded that laboratory studies of lymphocyte mitogen response could help contribute towards better management of patients receiving levamisole therapy [59].
Goebel et al. [60]	Goebel et al. reported on levamisole-induced immunostimulation in spondylarthropathies [60]. Goebel et al. concluded that levamisole might affect on defective immunoregulation in spondylarthropathies and, by improving the clinical conditions, led to a change in the course of this disease [60].
Fostiropoulos et al. [61]	Fostiropoulos et al. reported on once weekly administration of levamisole in rheumatoid arthritis [61]. Fostiropoulos et al. reported that once weekly was as effective as 3-day-weekly administration of levamisole, but resulted in fewer side-effects [61].
Verhaegen et al. [62]	Verhaegen et al. reported on immunologic evaluation of rheumatoid arthritis and therapy with levamisole [62]. Verhaegen et al. said that levamisole could restore cell-mediated immune reactivity and modify the natural course of rheumatoid arthritis [62].
Rosenthal et al. [63]	Rosenthal et al. reported on immunotherapy with levamisole in rheumatic diseases [63]. Rosenthal et al. concluded that this treatment demonstrated some potential hazardous complications of the drug and required physical and laboratory examinations at short intervals [63].
Pinals et al. [64]	Pinals et al. reported on a double-blind comparison of high and low doses of levamisole in rheumatoid arthritis. Pinals et al. concluded that levamisole was effective [64].
Seki et al. [65]	Seki et al. studied on induction of E-rosette-promoting factor in human plasma by levamisole [65]. Seki et al. concluded that levamisole might mediate an increased secretion of humoral factor with E-rosette-promoting activity, even from such a rudimentary thymus as in the partial DiGeorge syndrome [65].
Skotnicki [66]	Skotnicki reported on agranulocytosis in patients with rheumatoid arthritis treated with levamisole [66].

Table 2. Important reports on antibody treatment

Authors	Details
Muhamuda et al. [67]	Muhamuda et al. reported on use of neutralizing murine monoclonal antibodies to rabies glycoprotein in passive immunotherapy against rabies [67]. Muhamuda et al. concluded that the new murine monoclonal antibodies were found to be 2,000 times more potent than commercial ERIG in terms of effective protein concentration and neutralizing titer [67].
Baba [68]	Baba reported on Effect of immunoglobulin therapy on blood viscosity and potential concerns of thromboembolism focusing of Kawasaki disease [68]. Baba said that although there was only a few epidemiological data as to the prevalence of thromboembolism associated with immunoglobulin therapy therapy, the occurrence of these complications should be taken into consideration [68].
Kuo et al. [69]	Kuo et al. said that patient characteristics and intravenous immunoglobulin product could affect eosinophils in Kawasaki disease [69].
Khan et al. [70]	Khan et al. said that both patient characteristics and intravenous immunoglobulin product-specific mechanisms could affect eosinophils in immunoglobulin-treated Kawasaki disease [70].
Moreno et al. [71]	Moreno et al. reported on coronary involvement in infants with Kawasaki disease treated with intravenous gamma-globulin [71]. Of interest, Moreno et al. observed a high rate of infants who developed coronary arterial complications, which is similar to the one reported in children who do not receive immunotherapy [71].
de Melker and Steyerberg [72]	de Melker and Steyerberg reported on function of tetanus immunoglobulin in case of injury [72].
Miranda-Filho Dde et al. [73]	Miranda-Filho Dde et al. reported on randomised controlled trial of tetanus treatment with antitetanus immunoglobulin by the intrathecal or intramuscular route [73]. Miranda-Filho Dde et al. concluded that patients treated with antitetanus immunoglobulin by the intrathecal route showed better clinical progression than those treated by the intramuscular route [73].

CYTOKINE TREATMENT

Cytokine treatment makes use of administration of cytokine for curative purpose. This is famous for a long time for many diseases. Good examples are hepatitis virus infections. Important interesting reports on cytokine treatment will be given as idea to the readers in Table 3.

Table 3. Important reports on cytokine treatment

Authors	Details
Hedegaard et al. [74]	Hedegaard et al. reported on the effect of beta-interferon (IFN) therapy on myelin basic protein-elicited CD4+ T cell proliferation and cytokine production in multiple sclerosis [74].
Hwang and Gausas [75]	Hwang and Gausas reported on arcoid-like granulomatous orbital inflammation induced by IFN-alpha treatment [75].
Eggermont et al. [76]	Eggermont et al. reported that adjuvant pegylated IFN alfa-2b for stage III melanoma had a significant, sustained effect on recurrence-free survival [76].
Badr et al. [77]	Badr et al. suggested that poly-functionality of HCV-specific T cells could be predictive of the outcome of acute HCV and that early therapeutic intervention, IFN-alpha, antiviral therapy, could reconstitute the pool of long-lived poly-functional memory T cells [77].
Bolewska et al. [78]	Bolewska et al. studied on IFN alpha, gamma, omega before and during treatment of chronic hepatitis C with pegylated interferon alpha and ribavirin [78]. Bolewska et al. found that there was no correlation in IFN alpha, gamma and omega concentrations with efficacy of antiviral treatment [78].
Adamek et al. [68]	Adamek et al. studied on long-term viral response to IFN alpha 2b plus ribavirin in chronic HCV patients during standard therapy

REFERENCES

[1] Neu HC. The role of cellular and humoral factors in infections. *Clin Haematol.* 1976 Jun;5(2):449-65.

[2] Colten HR, Einstein LP. Complement metabolism: cellular and humoral regulation. *Transplant Rev.* 1976;32:3-11.

[3] McMurry JA, Johansson BE, De Groot AS. A call to cellular & humoral arms: enlisting cognate T cell help to develop broad-spectrum vaccines against influenza A. *Hum Vaccin.* 2008 Mar-Apr;4(2):148-57.

[4] Singer JM. Immunology of bacterial and fungal infections. *Mt Sinai J Med.* 1977 Jan-Feb;44(1):60-72.

[5] Frøland SS. Interaction of microbial agents with the immune system during infectious disease. *Acta Otolaryngol Suppl.* 1984;407:14-22.

[6] Olinescu A. Immune mechanisms of antiviral, bacterial and parasitic protection. *Rev Ig Bacteriol Virusol Parazitol Epidemiol Pneumoftiziol Bacteriol Virusol Parazitol Epidemiol.* 1988 Jan-Mar;33(1):15-28.

[7] Martín Mateos MA. The immune response in pediatric infections. *An Esp Pediatr.* 1989 Sep;31 Suppl 38:20-4.

[8] Giełdanowski J, Tuszewska R. Modern views on the mechanism of immune processes: I. Morphological substrate, biochemistry, types and kinetics of immune reactions (author's transl). *Klin Oczna.* 1977 Jul;47(7):309-13.

[9] Schulte-Wissermann H, Gardilcic S. Fundamentals of immunotherapy. (author's transl). *Klin Padiatr.* 1981 Mar;193(2):57-62.

[10] Loisel-Meyer S, Foley R, Medin JA. Immuno-gene therapy approaches for cancer: from in vitro studies to clinical trials. *Front Biosci.* 2008 May 1;13:3202-14.

[11] Mimori T, Homma M. Immunomodulation and immunomodulators. *Nippon Rinsho.* 1981 Apr;39(4):1847-51.

[12] Abe T. Development and clinical use of chemical immunomodulators. *Nippon Rinsho.* 1981 Apr;39(4):1893-901.

[13] Mizushima Y.Immunomodulator (author's transl). *Ryumachi.* 1980 Feb;20(1):57-62.

[14] Wiwanitkit, V. Imiquimod: a new immunomodulatory drug. *Chula Med J* 2004 May; 48(5):325 – 38.

[15] Slade HB. Cytokine induction and modifying the immune response to human papilloma virus with imiquimod. *Eur J Dermatol* 1998 Oct-Nov; 8(7 Suppl):13 – 6.

[16] Edwards L. Imiquimod in clinical practice. *J Am Acad Dermatol.* 2000 Jul; 43(1 pt 2): S12-7.

[17] Maw RD. Treatment of anogenital warts. *Dermatol Clin* 1998 Oct; 16(4): 829 – 34.

[18] Zerr DM, Frenkel LM. Advances in antiviral therapy. *Curr Opin Pediatr* 1999 Feb; 11(1): 21 – 7.

[19] Buck HW. Imiquimod (Aldara cream). *Infect Dis Obstet Gynecol* 1998; 6(2): 49 – 51.

[20] Gross G. Therapy of human papillomavirus infection and associated epithelial tumors. *Intervirology* 1997; 40(5-6): 368 – 77.

[21] Edwards L, Ferenczy A, Eron L, Baker D, Owens ML, Fox TL, Hougham AJ, Schmitt KA. Selfadministered topical 5 % imiquimod cream for external anogenital warts. HPV Study Group. Human PapillomaVirus. *Arch Dermatol* 1998 Jan; 134(1): 25 – 30.

[22] Beutner KR, Ferenczy A. Therapeutic approaches to genital warts. *Am J Med* 1997 May 5; 102(5A): 28 – 37.

[23] Baker GE, Tyring SK. Therapeutic approaches to papillomavirus infections. *Dermatol Clin* 1997 Apr; 15(2): 331 – 40.

[24] Memar OM, Tyring SK. Antiviral agents in dermatology: current status and future prospects. *Int J Dermatol* 1995 Sep; 34(9): 597 – 606.

[25] Arany I, Tyring SK, Brysk MM, Stanley MA, Tomai MA, Miller RL, Smith MH, McDermott DJ, Slade HB. Correlation between pretreatment levels of interferon response genes and clinical responses to an immune response modifier (Imiquimod) in genital warts. *Antimicrob Agents Chemother* 2000 Jul; 44(7):1869 – 73.

[26] Manlove-Simmons JM, Zaher FM, Tomai M, Gonik B, Svinarich DM. Effect of imiquimod on cytokine induction in first trimester trophoblasts. *Infect Dis Obstet Gynecol* 2000; 8(2): 105 – 11.

[27] Bottrel RL, Yang YL, Levy DE, Tomai M, Reis LF. The immune response modifier imiquimod requires STAT-1 for induction of interferon, interferon-stimulated genes, and interleukin-6. *Antimicrob Agents Chemother* 1999 Apr; 43(4): 856 – 61.

[28] Wagner TL, Ahonen CL, Couture AM, Gibson SJ, Miller RL, Smith RM, Reiter MJ, Vasilakos JP, Tomai MA. Modulation of TH1 and TH2 cytokine production with the immune response modifiers, R-848 and imiquimod. *Cell Immunol* 1999 Jan; 191(1): 10 – 9.

[29] Imbertson LM, Beaurline JM, Couture AM, Gibson SJ, Smith RM, Miller RL, Reiter MJ, Wagner TL, Tomai MA. Cytokine induction in hairless mouse and rat skin after topical application of the immune response modifiers imiquimod and S-28463. *J Invest Dermatol* 1998 May; 110(5): 734 – 9.

[30] Wagner TL, Horton VL, Carlson GL, Myhre PE, Gibson SJ, Imbertson LM, Tomai MA. Induction of cytokines in cynomolgus monkeys by the immune response modifiers, imiquimod, S-27609 and S-28463. *Cytokine* 1997 Nov; 9(11): 837 – 45.

[31] Fujisawa H, Shivji GM, Kondo S, Wang B, Tomai MA, Miller RL, Sauder DN. Effect of a novel topical immunomodulator, S-28463, on keratinocyte cytokine gene expression and production. *J Interferon Cytokine* Res 1996 Jul; 16(7): 555 – 9.

[32] Karaca K, Sharma JM, Tomai MA, Miller RL. In vivo and In vitro interferon induction in chickens by S - 28828, an imidazoquinolinamine immunoenhancer. *J Interferon Cytokine Res* 1996 Apr; 16(4): 327 – 32.

[33] Tomai MA, Gibson SJ, Imbertson LM, Miller RL, Myhre PE, Reiter MJ, Wagner TL, Tamulinas CB, Beaurline JM, Gerster JF. Immunomodulating and antiviral activities of the imidazoquinoline S-28463. *Antiviral Res* 1995 Nov; 28(3): 253 – 64.

[34] Testerman TL, Gerster JF, Imbertson LM, Reiter MJ, Miller RL, Gibson SJ, Wagner TL, Tomai MA. Cytokine induction by the immunomodulators imiquimod and S-27609. *J Leukoc Bio*l 1995 Sep; 58(3): 365 – 72.

[35] Gibson SJ, Imbertson LM, Wagner TL, Testerman TL, Reiter MJ, Miller RL, Tomai MA. Cellular requirements for cytokine production in response to the immunomodulators imiquimod and S-27609. *J Interferon Cytokine Res* 1995 Jun; 15(6): 537 – 45.

[36] Weeks CE, Gibson SJ. Induction of interferon and other cytokines by imiquimod and its hydroxylated metabolite R-842 in human blood cells in vitro. *J Interferon Res* 1994 Apr; 14(2): 81 – 5.

[37] Kono T, Kondo S, Pastore S, Shivji GM, Tomai MA, Mckenzie RC, Sauder DN. Effects of a novel topical immunomodulator, imiquimod, on keratinocyte cytokine gene expression. *Lymphokine Cytokine Res* 1994 Apr; 13(2) 71 – 6.

[38] Reiter MJ, Testerman TL, Miller RL, Weeks CE, Tomai MA. Cytokine induction in mice by the immunomodulator imiquimod. *J Leukoc Biol* 1994 Feb; 55(2): 234 – 40.

[39] Edwards L, Ferenczy A, Eron L, Baker D, Owens ML, Fox TL, Hougham AJ, Schmitt KA. Selfadministered topical 5 % imiquimod cream for external anogenital warts. HPV Study Group. Human PapillomaVirus. *Arch Dermatol* 1998 Jan; 134(1): 25 - 30.

[40] Maitland JE, Maw R. An audit of patients who have received imiquimod cream 5% for the treatment of anogenital warts. *Int J STD AIDS* 2000 Apr; 11(4): 268 – 70.

[41] Syed TA, Ahmadpour OA, Ahmad SA, Ahmad SH. Management of female genital warts with an analog of imiquimod 2% in cream: a randomized, double-blind, placebo-controlled study. *J Dermatol* 1998 Jul; 25(7): 429 – 33.

[42] Beutner KR, Spruance SL, Hougham AJ, Fox TL, Owens ML, Douglas JM Jr. Treatment of genital warts with an immune-response modifier (imiquimod). *J Am Acad Dermatol* 1998 Feb; 38(2 pt 1): 230 – 9.

[43] Beutner KR, Ferenczy A. Therapeutic approaches to genital warts. *Am J Med* 1997 May 5; 102(5A): 28 – 37.

[44] Apgar BS. Changes in strategies for human papillomavirus genital disease. *Am Fam Physician* 1997 Apr; 55(5): 1545 – 6.

[45] Baker GE, Tyring SK. Therapeutic approaches to papillomavirus infections. *Dermatol Clin* 1997 Apr;15(2): 331 – 40.

[46] 34. Langley PC, Richwald GA, Smith MH. Modeling the impact of treatment options in genital warts: patient-applied versus physicianadministered therapies. *Clin Ther* 1999 Dec; 21(12): 2143 – 55.

[47] Symoens J. Immunopharmacology of levamisole. *Z Hautkr*. 1979 May 1;54(9):394-402.

[48] Senn JS, Lai CC, Price GB. Levamisole: evidence for activity on human haemopoietic progenitor cells. *Br J Cancer*. 1980 Jan;41(1):40-6.

[49] Amery WK, Gough DA. Levamisole and immunotherapy: some theoretic and practical considerations and their relevance to human disease. *Oncology*. 1981;38(3):168-81.

[50] Smogorzewska E. Levamisole as an immunostimulating factor. *Probl Med Wieku Rozwoj*. 1979;8:56-62.

[51] Chumakova MM. Various aspects of the mechanism of action of levamisole. *Ter Arkh*. 1978;50(9):146-53

[52] Sakharchuk II, Skakal'skaia LM. Pharmacological and immunotherapeutic properties of levamisole (a review of the literature). *Vrach Delo*. 1982 Aug;(8):4-8.

[53] Renoux G. The general immunopharmacology of levamisole. *Drugs*. 1980 Aug;20(2):89-99.

[54] Levy J. Levamisole and cellular immunity in rheumatoid arthritis--clinical and laboratory correlates. *J Rheumatol Suppl*. 1978;4:63-70.

[55] Taki HN, Schwartz SA. reportedLevamisole as an immunopotentiator for T cell deficiency. *Immunopharmacol Immunotoxicol*. 1994 May;16(2):129-37.

[56] Rosenthal M, Trabert U, Müller W. The effect of Levamisole on peripheral blood lymphocyte subpopulations in patients with rheumatoid arthritis and ankylosing spondylitis. *Clin Exp Immunol*. 1976 Sep;25(3):493-6.

[57] Runge LA, Rynes RI. Balancing effectiveness and toxicity of levamisole in the treatment of rheumatoid arthritis. *Clin Exp Rheumatol*. 1983 Apr-Jun;1(2):125-31.

[58] Giulling EV, Kravchuk GP, Kazirchuk VE, Maksiuk LV, Zabolotnyĭ DI. Prediction of the effectiveness of levamisole immunotherapy by the sensitivity of blood lymphocytes to the drug. *Vrach Delo*. 1984 Nov;(11):38-42

[59] Levy J. Correlations of clinical and laboratory effects of treatment with levamisole in autoimmune disease. *Cancer Treat Rep*. 1978 Nov;62(11):1715-9.

[60] Goebel KM, Goebel FD, Schubotz R, Hahn E, Neurath F. Levamisole-induced immunostimulation in spondylarthropathies. *Lancet*. 1977 Jul 30;2(8031):214-7.

[61] Fostiropoulos GA, Zissis NP, Marketos G. Once weekly administration of levamisole in rheumatoid arthritis. *Clin Invest Med*. 1982;5(4):255-8.

[62] Verhaegen H, de Cree J, de Cock W, Schuermans Y, Engels M, Sonck W. Immunologic evaluation of rheumatoid arthritis and therapy with levamisole. *Biomedicine*. 1977 Jul;26(4):283-91.

[63] Rosenthal M, Trabert U, Müller W. Immunotherapy with levamisole in rheumatic diseases. *Scand J Rheumatol*. 1976;5(4):216-20.

[64] Pinals RS, Robertson F, Blechman WJ. A double-blind comparison of high and low doses of levamisole in rheumatoid arthritis. *J Rheumatol*. 1981 Nov-Dec;8(6):949-51.

[65] Seki H, Yokoi T, Kubo M, Moriya N, Miyawaki T, Nagaoki T, Miura M, Taniguchi N. Induction of E-rosette-promoting factor in human plasma by levamisole: an assessment in a patient with partial DiGeorge syndrome. *Scand J Immunol*. 1982 Feb;15(2):141-8.

[66] Skotnicki AB. Agranulocytosis in patients with rheumatoid arthritis treated with levamisole--mechanism and prevention. *Przegl Lek*. 1982;39(9):613-6.

[67] Muhamuda K, Madhusudana SN, Ravi V. Use of neutralizing murine monoclonal antibodies to rabies glycoprotein in passive immunotherapy against rabies. *Hum Vaccin*. 2007 Sep-Oct;3(5):192-5.

[68] Baba R. Effect of immunoglobulin therapy on blood viscosity and potential concerns of thromboembolism, especially in patients with acute Kawasaki disease. *Recent Patents Cardiovasc Drug Discov*. 2008 Jun;3(2):141-4.

[69] Kuo HC, Wang CL, Wang L, Yu HR, Yang KD. Patient characteristics and intravenous immunoglobulin product may affect eosinophils in Kawasaki disease. *Pediatr Allergy Immunol*. 2008 Mar;19(2):184-5.

[70] Khan S, Doré PC, Sewell WA. Both patient characteristics and IVIG product-specific mechanisms may affect eosinophils in immunoglobulin-treated Kawasaki disease. *Pediatr Allergy Immunol*. 2008 Mar;19(2):186-7.

[71] Moreno N, Méndez-Echevarría A, de Inocencio J, Del Castillo F, Baquero-Artigao F, García-Miguel MJ, de José MI, Aracil J. Coronary involvement in infants with Kawasaki disease treated with intravenous gamma-globulin. *Pediatr Cardiol*. 2008 Jan;29(1):31-5. Epub 2007 Oct 5.

[72] de Melker HE, Steyerberg EW. Function of tetanus immunoglobulin in case of injury: administration often unnecessary. *Ned Tijdschr Geneeskd*. 2004 Feb 28;148(9):429-33.

[73] Miranda-Filho Dde B, Ximenes RA, Barone AA, Vaz VL, Vieira AG, Albuquerque VM. Randomised controlled trial of tetanus treatment with antitetanus immunoglobulin by the intrathecal or intramuscular route. *BMJ*. 2004 Mar 13;328(7440):615.

[74] Hedegaard CJ, Krakauer M, Bendtzen K, Sørensen PS, Sellebjerg F, Nielsen CH. The effect of beta-interferon therapy on myelin basic protein-elicited CD4+ T cell proliferation and cytokine production in multiple sclerosis. *Clin Immunol*. 2008 Jul 22. [Epub ahead of print]

[75] Hwang CJ, Gausas RE. Sarcoid-like granulomatous orbital inflammation induced by interferon-alpha treatment. *Ophthal Plast Reconstr Surg*. 2008 Jul-Aug;24(4):311-3.

[76] Eggermont AM, Suciu S, Santinami M, Testori A, Kruit WH, Marsden J, Punt CJ, Salès F, Gore M, Mackie R, Kusic Z, Dummer R, Hauschild A, Musat E, Spatz A,

Keilholz U; EORTC Melanoma Group. Adjuvant therapy with pegylated interferon alfa-2b versus observation alone in resected stage III melanoma: final results of EORTC 18991, a randomised phase III trial. *Lancet.* 2008 Jul 12;372(9633):117-26.

[77] Badr G, Bédard N, Abdel-Hakeem MS, Trautmann L, Willems B, Villeneuve JP, Haddad EK, Sékaly RP, Bruneau J, Shoukry NH. Early Interferon Therapy for HCV Rescues Poly-functional long-lived CD8+ Memory T Cells. *J Virol.* 2008 Jul 30. [Epub ahead of print]

[78] Bolewska B, Czajka A, Moczko J, Juszczyk J. Interferon alpha, gamma, omega before and during treatment of chronic hepatitis C with pegylated interferon alpha and ribavirin. *Przegl Epidemiol.* 2007;61(4):755-63

[79] Adamek A, Adamek J, Juszczyk J, Bereszyńska I. Long-term viral response to interferon alpha 2b plus ribavirin in chronic hepatitis C patients during standard therapy. *Przegl Epidemiol.* 2007;61(4):765-70.

Chapter XII

THERAPEUTIC VACCINATION

INTRODUCTION TO VACCINE [1-15]

Vaccine is a specific important tool in medicine. Due to the principle of immunity, human beings require immune to defend any alien foreign bodies. However, immunity cannot be functional if there is no previous exposure. This means it has to be a memory before immune generation or the human beings must experience previous foreign bodies' invasion. However, in some cases, immunity is slightly generated and cannot fight with external invasion of align foreign bodies and this brings mortality and morbidity. Therefore, simulating the invasion of align foreign bodies to prepare for real invasion is needed and very useful. This is the concept of vaccination. Vaccination is defined as a primary prevention. Vaccine can prevent before real existence. Vaccine is a mode of simulating interaction as previously described.

Vaccination is classified as an active immunization. This means tit makes uses of human beings physiological process to create immune by itself. There are several vaccine at present. Recommendation for vaccination might be different in different settings. Expanded Program on Immunization (EPI) is the basic public health one in all countries. With use of vaccine, controls of many infectious diseases are feasible. Pox is an example of infectious disease that can be controlled by vaccine. This infection is already got rid of by succeed in global vaccination. The presently widely used vaccine include rabies vaccine, measles vaccine, rubella vaccine, Japanese encephalitis vaccine, hepatitis B vaccine, hepatitis A vaccine, influenza vaccine, varicella vaccine, pneumococcal vaccine, pertussis vaccine, diphtheria vaccine, BCG and toxiod. However, at present, there are attempts to develop more vaccines for real clinical usage/. This is the aim of preventive medicine. In addition, there are attempts to develop vaccine for expanded usefulness. This is the origin of therapeutic vaccine. This is the new trend to use vaccine as treatment tool. This is classified as immunotherapy. The details of this new way of immunotherapy will be further detailed and discussed in this chapter. To produce a therapeutic vaccine, it might be a basic knowledge on biotechnology and immunology. More details on this item can be seen in this chapter.

How can Therapeutic Vaccine Act? [1-15]

Therapeutic vaccinations is used for treatment, therefore, it must have the property for curative purpose. The concept for therapeutic vaccine makes uses of basic immunology principle and how the therapeutic vaccine can act can be explained by basic principles of vaccination. Vaccination is basically administered among recipients aiming at active immune generation. This means the vaccine itself stimulates the immune system of the recipient to generate immunity that can be used for further defensive mechanism. This can be also applied for the case of therapeutic vaccination. For therapeutic vaccination, the vaccine is also applied aiming at stimulation of active immunity generation, however, it is administered when the recipient already has got disease. Other processes are same as classical vaccination. Producing of immunity is the tool for treatment of pathological disorders and this is the aim of application of therapeutic vaccination as previously said. This is the concept that alerts medical scientists to find new therapeutic vaccines, to design and to launch the new ones for real clinical usage. Some important examples and an example on specific therapeutic vaccination research will be given to the readers in this chapter to make better understand on this topic.

Immunomics

Immumomics is the modern omics science. Routinely, the outstanding diversity of immune system components together with the complex apperance of the regulatory pathways and network-type interactions come immunology a combinatorial science [16-17]. Immunomics starts from immunoinformatics [18]. Computational analysis is an essential element of immunology research with a major role of immunoinformatics being the management and analysis of immunological data [16]. More advanced analyses of the immune system making use of computational models typically involve conversion of an immunological question to a computational problem, followed by solving of the computational problem and translation of these results into biologically meaningful solutions [16]. Main immunoinformatics developments cover immunological databases, sequence analysis, structure modeling, mathematical modeling of the immune system, simulation of laboratory experiments, statistical support for immunological experimentation and immunogenomics [16]. Basically immunoinformatics will look at immunological databases, antigen processing and presentation, immunogenomics, host-pathogen interactions, and mathematical modeling of the immune system [19-20]. Human and mouse genome and transcriptome projects have broadened the field of immunogenetics beyond the traditional study of the genetics and evolution of MHC, TCR and Ig loci into the modern interdisciplinary area of immunomics [20]. Basically, a high-throughput approach permitting correlation between newly discovered genes and functional properties of their protein products has yet to be developed [21]. To show relationships between tens of thousands of genes and their cognate proteins, modern interdisciplinary technologies need to emerge [21]. Immunomics is the work of the molecular functions associated with all immune-related coding and non-coding mRNA transcripts [20]. It is noted that advance techniques in immunomics will foster development of new diagnostic, immune-based treatment, and vaccine programs [22]. Aims of present molecular epidemiology study on infectious diseases and cancer [23-26] are closely related to the field of immunomics. The aim of these researches was a) to molecularly determine the circulating pathogenic strains, b) to follow up alterations in regulatory and coding sequences over time and c) to choose a representative pathogenic strain as template for vaccine development. Circulating pathogenic strains can be detected by the previously mentioned biotechnology technique. Persistence of many molecular forms and changing proportions over time can be imagined. Phylogenetic analysis of sequences to identify molecular forms, their relationships, proportions at each visit, and fluctuations over time can be useful for researching alterations. Relied on extensive sequence analysis of various pathogen isolates and molecular cloning of selected virtually full length genomes, necessarily dominating pathogen types can be found to circulate throughout a setting. The most identified type with minimal genetic drift can be chose as template for the design of vaccines.

DEVELOPMENT OF NEW VACCINE

Development of new vaccine is the new way for non curative malignancy and new emerging infectious diseases prevention and treatment. New vaccines can be searched using a wide range of technologies, yielding items ranging from nonspecific immunostimulants through to highly technical peptide- and DNA-based candidates [27]. There are several technical challenges involved in even the most basic decisions in vaccine development, such as the choosing of antigen, formulation, adjuvant, route of delivery and schedule [27]. Routinely, vaccine development includes determining the epitope of targeted protein, development of recombinant and test for its efficacy. Routinely, this process starts from in vitro works to in vivo researches (from animal model to human clinical researches). Paul et al. said that the same vaccination strategies applied for prophylactic vaccinations against infectious diseases could not necessarily be applied for therapeutic cancer vaccination [28]. They also said that cancer patients were commonly immunosuppressed and most cancer-associated antigens were self-antigens, making it an important challenge to vaccinate patients against a cancer-associated antigen [28]. The aim of new vaccine is to evoke active immunity in the vaccinees. Basically, both humoral and cellular immune responses are focused. Humoral immune response assist destroy malignany cells via circulating antibodies and cellular immune response assist destroy malignant cells via cytotoxic and cytokine processes. In addition to the classical immunological technique, with advent in bioinformatics, development of modern cancer vaccine can be done by advanced in silico techniques.

1. Finding Epitope

To find a peptide candidate for a vaccine, the starting point is to find appropriate epitpes. Different means for epitope mapping are available at present [29]. It should be noted that synthetic peptide vaccines aiming at the induction of a protective response against malignant disorders are widely trialed but despite their success in animal experiments they do not yet live up to their promise in humans [30]. Mapping for possible epitopes seems to be a difficult step. The evidence accumulating from several recent studies points to a broader range of targets recognized than previously imagined, in terms of both numbers and characteristics of the targeted antigens [31]. Also, multiple studies reveal a substantial variation in the targets recognized in different human individuals [31]. To solve the problem of heterogenicity, many new computational tools are developed for finding of probable candidate vaccine epitopes. Prediction of both T cell and B cell epitopes for further cancer vaccine development can be easily done. For example, Wiwanitkit used a computational technique to detect T-cell epitopes for a melanoma vaccine by an immunomics technique [32]. Wiwanitkit also performed another similar study to predicted B-cell epitopes of HER-2 oncoprotein by a bioinformatics mean to be a clue for breast cancer vaccine development [33].

2. Establishment of new Vaccine Recombinant

Establishment of new vaccine recombinant from alternative epitope is the additional next process. This can be done based on roles of artificial genetic recombinant. To develop modern genetic recombinant, advanced gene delivery and transfer technique can be used. Of several techniques, gene transfer by virus or transfection in the most widely applied. For example, Trevor el al reported their successful work in transduction of human dendritic cells with a recombinant modified vaccinia Ankara virus encoding MUC1 and IL-2 [34]. In addition to the basic artificial genetic recombinant generation, it can be performed by in silico mutating mean. An in silico template for new vaccine recombinant can easily available by classical mutation in sequence coding.

3. Trial for new Vaccine Efficacy

Trial for the vaccine efficacy is the last step of vaccine development. This can be done as the mentioned process in the heading of research into cancer vaccine. Clinical trials should be done prior to real generalization of the new vaccine. In order to decrease the long phase of clinical trial, the applied usage of advanced medical informatics technology, gene ontology [35], can assist predict the function or phenotypic expression of new developed vaccine. Schonbach et al. noted that support of vaccine development through textmining needed the timely development of domain-specific extraction rules for full-text articles, and a knowledge model for epitope-related information [36]. In order to test the new vaccine efficacy, another advanced bioinformatics technique can be helpful. To test the modern recombinant, gene ontology can be served. Routinely, function and other information concerning genes are to be captured, made accessible to biologists or structured in a computable form as a new sight [37]. Gene ontology is the modern "logy" for this propose. Gene ontology is a scientific word applied to describe the biology of a gene product in any organism. It also implies the description of the molecular functions of gene products, the corresponding placement in and as cellular components, and the participation in biological processes [38]. Since much of biology works by applying previously known knowledge to an unknown entity, the application of a set of axioms that will bring knowledge and the complex biological information stored in bioinformatics databases are necessary [38]. These often need addition of knowledge to specify and constrain the values held in that database and a track of capturing knowledge within bioinformatics applications and databases is the use of ontologies [38]. Since the early of this century, the Gene Ontology (GO) Consortium has been detected. The aim of the GO Consortium is to bring and create a framework for both the description and the organization of such information [39]. The Gene Ontology (GO) project find the way to provide a set of structured vocabularies for specific biological domains that can be applied to describe gene products in any organism [40]. The research includes building three extensive ontologies to describe molecular function, biological process, and cellular component, and giving a community database resource that supports the use of these ontologies [40]. In the present day, gene ontology can also be used for advance research in medicine and can be useful for testing of new vaccine.

Application of Immunonics for Therapeutic Vaccine Research

As previously mentioned, immunomics can be applied for therapeutic vaccine research. BCG and its effect on prostate cancer antigen 1 by a gene ontology study is hereby presented as an example.

A. Introduction

Prostate cancer is an important cancer in male population. It is the most common cancer in male populations in many parts of the world. It is a slowing growing deadly cancer with only a few signs and symptoms in the early stage of disease [41]. Causes of the disease are essentially not known, although hormonal factors are involved, and diet may increase an indirect influence; some genes, potentially involved in hereditary prostate cancer (HPC) have been identified [42]. A suspect of prostate cancer may derive from increased serum prostate-specific antigen (PSA) values and/or a suspicious digital rectal examination (DRE) finding [42]. However, there is insufficient evidence to either help or refute the routine use of mass, selective or opportunistic screening compared to no screening for reducing prostate cancer fatality [43].

Identifying the genetic factors involved in prostate carcinogenesis is critical. A gene, designated prostate cancer antigen-1 shows high mRNA expression in prostate cancer [44]. Prostate cancer antigen 1 becomes a specific new marker for prostate cancer. In addition, Prostate cancer antigen 1 may also serve as a therapeutic target molecule for prostate cancer [44]. For treatment, prostatectomy is a standard therapeutic method. However, there are other additional treatments. BCG (Bacillus of Calmette Guerin) has been in use for more than 20 years and is currently the most active agent for superficial bladder cancer therapy [45].

Intravesical BCG therapy is effective in prophylaxis after transurethral resection of papillary tumours and in the therapeutic process of carcinoma in situ (cis) [45].

To study the interaction between BCG treatment and prostate cancer antigen 1, the new development in bioinformatics can be applied. Here, the author used a new gene ontology technology to predict the change in molecular function resulting from the combination between BCG and prostate cancer antigen 1.

B. Materials and Methods

For getting the sequence, the database PubMed was used for information mining of the amino acid sequence for BCG and prostate cancer antigen 1. Prediction of molecular function and biological process was further done. The author performs prediction of molecular function and biological process of BCG and prostate cancer antigen 1 using a novel gene ontology prediction tool, GoFigure [46]. GoFigure is an computational algorithm tool which is recently used in gene ontology [46]. The tool accepts an input DNA or protein sequence, and uses BLAST to identify homologous sequences in GO annotated databases [46]. The approach is to apply a BLAST search to identify homologs in public databases that have been annotated with gene ontology terms [47]. These terms include: SwissProt, Flybase (Drosophila), the Saccharomyces Genome Database (SGD), Mouse Genome Informatics (MGI) and Wormbase (nematode) [47]. The contents of the results will show outcomes for molecular function as well as biological process of the studied protein [47]. The prediction of molecular function were presented and compared.

C. Results

From searching of the database, sequence of BCG and prostate cancer antigen 1 can be got and used for further study. Using GoFigure server, the molecular functions in BCG, prostate cancer antigen 1 and combination between BCG and prostate cancer antigen 1 are predicted. The molecular functions in a combination between BCG and prostate cancer antigen 1 is presented in Figure 1.

D. Discussion

New developments have forced a re-evaluation of our understanding on cancer treatment. Immunological treatment is the novel mode of cancer therapy. For prostate cancer, BCG was introduced to be a tool of treatment for a long time. BCG is established for localized bladder cancer and many experimental immunotherapies are under evaluating processes [47]. Saitoh et al. found that reduction of telomerase activity is related to the mechanism of BCG effects [48]. Here, the author studied the change in molecular function of prostate cancer antigen 1 treated with BCG. The gene ontology technique is used. This technique is a new concept and used in some recent molecular biological studies [49-50]. Of interest, the combination between both molecules affect majorly on cytoskeletal system. This finding can be a good explanation for the effectiveness of BCG in treatment of prostate cancer. Indeed, the cytoskeletal is the present target for treatment of solid tumor and anticancer drug development presently tacks on cytoskeletal stabilization [51]. However, further experimental studies are needed before making a conclusion on this topic. The finding in this study is not only supports the previous knowledge on BCG but also gives the new view on the therapy of prostate cancer.

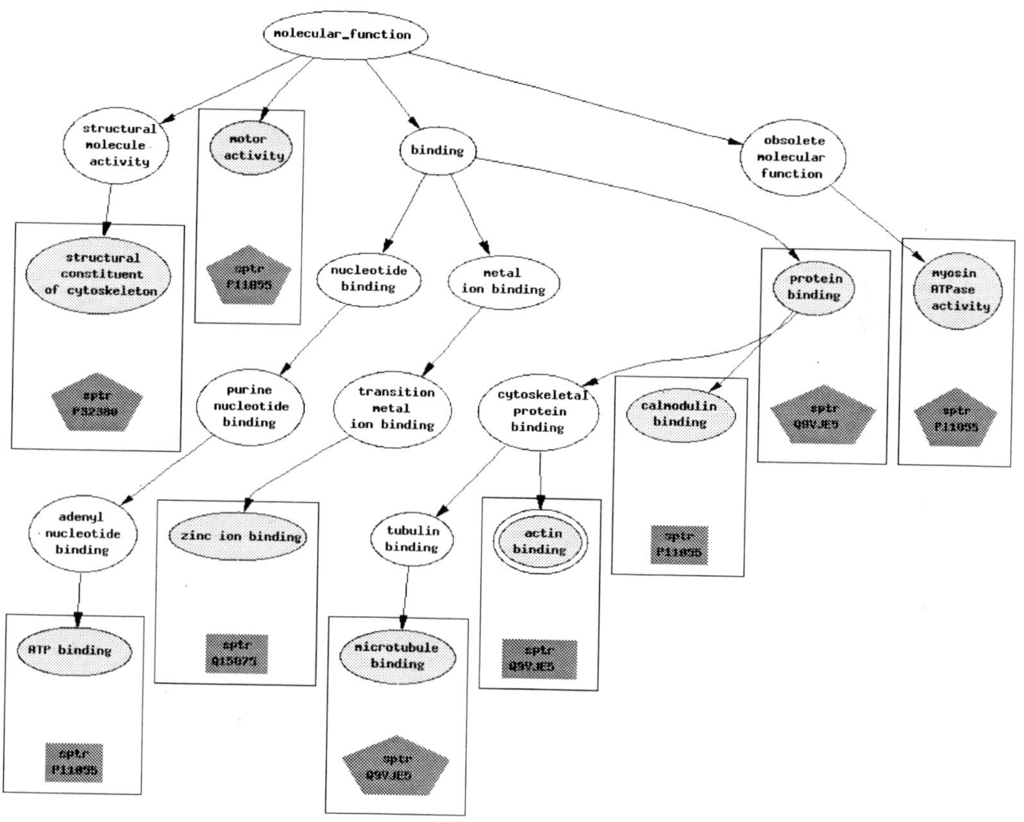

Figure 1. The molecular functions in a combination between BCG and prostate cancer antigen.

Therapeutic Vaccine at Present

We can observe that the therapeutic vaccine is aiming at curative of non curable disease especially cancers. There are many ongoing researches on this area.

The author hereby presents examples of such researches in Table 1.

Table 1. Application of immunomics for therapeutic vaccine research

Authors	Details
Huebener et al. [52]	Huebener et al. reported for the first time effective therapeutic vaccination followed by suppression of established spontaneous neuroblastoma metastases applying a tyrosine hydroxylase (TH) DNA minigene vaccine [52]. Huebener et al. Showed effective therapeutic vaccination against neuroblastoma with a novel rationally designed TH minigene vaccine without induction of autoimmunity giving an important baseline for future clinical application of this strategy [52].
Wheeler et al. [53]	Wheeler et al. said that therapeutic vaccination was an intriguing additional therapy for glioblastoma multiforme [53]. Wheeler et al. firstly reported a progressive correlation between cancer clinical outcome and T-cell responsiveness after therapeutic vaccination in humans and the first tracing of such correlation to therapeutically exploitable tumor alteration [53].
Wansley et al. [54]	Wansley et al. reported that vaccination with a recombinant *Saccharomyces cerevisiae* expressing a tumor antigen could break immune tolerance and led to therapeutic antitumor responses [54]. In this work, Wansley et al. found that vaccination with a heat-killed recombinant yeast expressing the tumor-associated antigen CEA could induce CEA-specific immune responses, decrease tumor burden, and expand overall survival in CEA-Tg mice [54].
Quenelle et al. [55]	Quenelle et al. reported on effect of an immune enhancer, GPI-0100, on vaccination with live attenuated herpes simplex virus (HSV) type 2 or glycoprotein D on genital HSV-2 infections of guinea pigs [55].
Smahel et al. [56]	Smahel et al. reported on enhancement of T cell-mediated and humoral immunity of beta-glucuronidase-based DNA vaccines against HPV16 E7 oncoprotein [56]. Smahel et al. reported that this mean led to the predominant localization of the fusion protein in the endoplasmic reticulum and enhancement of CD8+ T-cell response, while antibody production was decreased [56].
Park et al. [57]	Park et al. reported that codelivery of PEG-IFN-alpha might inhibit HCV DNA vaccine-induced T cell responses but not humoral responses in African green monkeys [57].
Mehendale et al. [58]	Mehendale et al. reported on a phase 1 study to evaluate the safety and immunogenicity of a recombinant HIV type 1 subtype C adeno-associated virus vaccine [58].
Romero [59]	Romero reported on current state of vaccine therapies in non-small-cell lung cancer [59]. Romero said that the vaccines usually tacked two main antigens widely expressed in lung carcinomas: melanoma-associated antigen 3, a cancer testis antigen; and mucin 1, an antigen overexpressed in a largely deglycosylated form in advanced tumors [59].
Zhang et al. [60]	Zhang et al. reported on cloning and expression of Vibrio harveyi OmpK* and GAPDH* genes and their potential application as vaccines in large yellow croakers *Pseudosciaena crocea* [60].
Cipriani et al. [61]	Cipriani et al. mentioned for the potential of genetic vaccines for the therapeutic treatment of malignancies and suggested probable predictive biomarkers to be further validated in the clinic for the follow-up of vaccinated cancerous patients [61].
Waites et al. [62]	Waites et al. reported on revaccination of adults with spinal cord injury using the 23-valent pneumococcal polysaccharide vaccine [62].
Rossi et al. [63]	Rossi et al. reported that allogeneic melanoma vaccine expressing alphaGal epitopes could bring antitumor immunity to autologous antigens in mice without signs of toxicity [63].
Amato et al. [64]	Amato et al. reported on an attenuated vaccinia virus, modified vaccinia Ankara engineered to deliver the tumor antigen 5T4 (TroVax) [64].
Redman et al. [65]	Redman et al. reported on phase Ib trial assessing autologous, tumor-pulsed dendritic cells as a vaccine administered with or without IL-2 in patients with metastatic melanoma [65]. Redman et al. found that the studied autologous tumor lysate-pulsed DC vaccine with or without IL-2 was well tolerated and immunogenic but failed to induce clinical response in patients with advanced melanoma [65].
Ge et al. [66]	Ge et al. reported on the antitumor immune responses induced by nanoemulsion-encapsulated MAGE1-HSP70/SEA complex protein vaccine following peroral administration route [66].

REFERENCES

[1] Minkoff NB. Multiple vaccines: how do we choose? *J Manag Care Pharm.* 2007 Sep;13(7 Suppl B):S16-20.

[2] Cannon HE. Pharmacy management of vaccines. *J Manag Care Pharm.* 2007 Sep;13(7 Suppl B):S7-11.

[3] Armstrong EP. Economic benefits and costs associated with target vaccinations. *J Manag Care Pharm.* 2007 Sep;13(7 Suppl B):S12-5.

[4] Holmgren J. Mucosal immunity and vaccination. *FEMS Microbiol Immunol.* 1991 Dec;4(1):1-9

[5] Walker RI. New strategies for using mucosal vaccination to achieve more effective immunization. *Vaccine.* 1994 Apr;12(5):387-400.

[6] Czerkinsky C, Quiding M, Eriksson K, Nordström I, Lakew M, Weneräs C, Kilander A, Björck S, Svennerholm AM, Butcher E, et al.. Induction of specific immunity at mucosal surfaces: prospects for vaccine development. *Adv Exp Med Biol.* 1995;371B:1409-16.

[7] Zinkernagel RM. On natural and artificial vaccinations. *Annu Rev Immunol.* 2003;21:515-46

[8] Arribas JL, Hernández-Navarrete MJ, Solano VM. Adult vaccination update. *Enferm Infecc Microbiol Clin.* 2004 Jun-Jul;22(6):342-54.

[9] Beytout J, Laurichesse H. Adult immunization in France: an update. *Rev Prat.* 2004 Mar 15;54(5):499-505

[10] Zimmerman RK, Middleton DB, Smith NJ. Vaccines for persons at high risk due to medical conditions, occupation, environment, or lifestyle, 2003. *J Fam Pract.* 2003 Jan;52(1 Suppl):S22-35.

[11] de Miguel AG. Strategies of vaccination for adult population in Spain in the actuality. *An R Acad Nac Med (Madr).* 2006;123(1):175-94.

[12] Zimmerman RK, Ball JA. Adult vaccinations. *Prim Care.* 2001 Dec;28(4):763-90, vi.

[13] Zimmerman RK, Middleton DB. Vaccines for persons at high risk due to medical conditions, occupation, environment, or lifestyle, 2005. *J Fam Pract.* 2005 Jan;54(1 Suppl):S27-36.

[14] Menzies R, McIntyre P. Vaccine preventable diseases and vaccination policy for indigenous populations. *Epidemiol Rev.* 2006;28:71-80.

[15] Loutan L. Vaccination of the immunocompromised patient. *Biologicals.* 1997 Jun;25(2):231-6.

[16] Barata Rde C. The challenge of emergent diseases and the return to descriptive epidemiology. *Rev Saude Publica.* 1997 Oct;31(5):531-7.

[17] Maslow JN, Mulligan ME, Arbeit RD. Molecular epidemiology: application of contemporary techniques to the typing of microorganisms. *Clin Infect Dis.* 1993 Aug;17(2):153-62.

[18] Lo YM, Chan KC. Introduction to the polymerase chain reaction. *Methods Mol Biol.* 2006;336:1-10.

[19] Maule J. Pulsed-field gel electrophoresis. *Mol Biotechnol.* 1998 Apr;9(2):107-26.

[20] Trgovcevic Z. 50 years of molecular biology. *Lijec Vjesn.* 1994 Nov-Dec;116(11-12):315-8.

[21] Fleischmann RD, Adams MD, White O, Clayton RA, Kirkness EF, Kerlavage AR, Bult CJ, Tomb JF, Dougherty BA, Merrick JM, et al.. Wole-genome random sequencing and assembly of Haemophilus influenzae Rd. *Science.* 1995 Jul 28;269(5223):496-512.

[22] Lewin R. National Academy looks at human genome project, sees progress. *Science.* 1987 Feb 13;235(4790):747-8.

[23] Foxman B, Riley L. Molecular epidemiology: focus on infection. *Am J Epidemiol.* 2001 Jun 15;153(12):1135-41.

[24] Lipuma JJ. Molecular tools for epidemiologic study of infectious diseases. *Pediatr Infect Dis J.* 1998 Aug;17(8):667-75.

[25] Riapis LA, Filatov NN, Salova NIa. Molecular epidemiology of infectious diseases. *Zh Mikrobiol Epidemiol Immunobiol.* 2003 Sep-Oct;(5):49-54.

[26] Tarasevich IV, Shaginyan IA, Mediannikov OY. Problems and perspectives of molecular epidemiology of infectious diseases. *Ann N Y Acad Sci.* 2003 Jun;990:751-6.

[27] Autret-Leca E, Jonville-Bera AP, Beau-Salinas F. Vaccines pharmacovigilance. *Rev Prat.* 2004 Mar 15;54(5):526-31.

[28] Paul S, Acres B, Limacher JM, Bonnefoy JY. Cancer vaccines: challenges and outlook in the field. *IDrugs.* 2007 May;10(5):324-8.

[29] Corradin G. Antigen processing and presentation. *Immunol Lett.* 1990 Aug;25(1-3):11-3.

[30] Bijker MS, Melief CJ, Offringa R, van der Burg SH. Design and development of synthetic peptide vaccines: past, present and future. *Expert Rev Vaccines.* 2007 Aug;6(4):591-603.

[31] Sette A, Peters B. Immune epitope mapping in the post-genomic era: lessons for vaccine development. *Curr Opin Immunol.* 2007 Feb;19(1):106-10.

[32] Wiwanitkit V. Finding a T-cell epitope for a melanoma vaccine by an immunomics technique. *Asian Pac J Cancer Prev.* 2006 Oct-Dec;7(4):659-60.

[33] Wiwanitkit V. Predicted B-cell epitopes of HER-2 oncoprotein by a bioinformatics method: a clue for breast cancer vaccine development. *Asian Pac J Cancer Prev.* 2007 Jan-Mar;8(1):137-8.

[34] Pecher G, Spahn G, Schirrmann T, Kulbe H, Ziegner M, Schenk JA, Sandig V. Mucin gene (MUC1) transfer into human dendritic cells by cationic liposomes and recombinant adenovirus. *Anticancer Res.* 2001 Jul-Aug;21(4A):2591-6.

[35] Thomas PD, Mi H, Lewis S. Ontology annotation: mapping genomic regions to biological function. *Curr Opin Chem Biol.* 2007 Feb;11(1):4-11.

[36] Schonbach C, Nagashima T, Konagaya A. Textmining in support of knowledge discovery for vaccine development. *Methods.* 2004 Dec;34(4):488-95.

[37] Ashburner M, Lewis S. On ontologies for biologists: the Gene Ontology--untangling the web. *Novartis Found Symp.* 2002; 247:66-80

[38] Takai T, Takagi T. Introduction to gene ontology. *Tanpakushitsu Kakusan Koso.* 2003; 48(1):79-85.

[39] Stevens R, Goble CA, Bechhofer S. Ontology-based knowledge representation for bioinformatics. *Brief. Bio*inform. 2000; 1(4):398-414.

[40] Gene Ontology Consortium. Creating the gene ontology resource: design and implementation. *Genome Res*. 2001; 11(8):1425-33.

[41] Prostate cancer: prevention and management of localized disease. *Nurse Pract*. 2006 Sep;31(9):14-29.

[42] Bracarda S, de Cobelli O, Greco C, Prayer-Galetti T, Valdagni R, Gatta G, de Braud F, Bartsch G. Cancer of the prostate. *Crit Rev Oncol Hematol*. 2005 Dec;56(3):379-96.

[43] Ilic D, O'Connor D, Green S, Wilt T. Screening for prostate cancer. *Cochrane Database Syst Rev*. 2006 Jul 19;3:CD004720.

[44] Konishi N, Nakamura M, Ishida E, Shimada K, Mitsui E, Yoshikawa R, Yamamoto H, Tsujikawa K. High expression of a new marker PCA-1 in human prostate carcinoma. *Clin Cancer Re*s. 2005 Jul 15;11(14):5090-7.

[45] Bassi P. BCG (Bacillus of Calmette Guerin) therapy of high-risk superficial bladder cancer. *Surg Oncol*. 2002 Jun;11(1-2):77-83.

[46] Kustner HG. Trends in four major communicable diseases. *S Afr Med J*. 1979;55:460-73.

[47] Totterman TH, Loskog A, Essand M. The immunotherapy of prostate and bladder cancer. *BJU Int*. 2005 Oct;96(5):728-35.

[48] Saitoh H, Mori K, Kudoh S, Itoh H, Takahashi N, Suzuki T. BCG effects on telomerase activity in bladder cancer cell lines. *Int J Clin Oncol*. 2002 Jun;7(3):165-70.

[49] Wiwanitkit V. Interaction between BRCA1 and human papilloma virus E7: an ontology study. *Arch Gynecol Obstet*. 2006;274:146-9.

[50] Tsai JR, Chong IW, Chen CC, Lin SR, Sheu CC, Hwang JJ. Mitogen-activated protein kinase pathway was significantly activated in human bronchial epithelial cells by nicotine. *DNA Cell Biol*. 2006;25:312-22.

[51] Ramaswamy B, Puhalla S. Docetaxel: a tubulin-stabilizing agent approved for the management of several solid tumors. *Drugs Today (Barc)*. 2006 Apr;42(4):265-79.

[52] Huebener N, Fest S, Strandsby A, Michalsky E, Preissner R, Zeng Y, Gaedicke G, Lode HN. A rationally designed tyrosine hydroxylase DNA vaccine induces specific antineuroblastoma immunity. *Mol Cancer Ther*. 2008 Jul;7(7):2241-51.

[53] Wheeler CJ, Black KL, Liu G, Mazer M, Zhang XX, Pepkowitz S, Goldfinger D, Ng H, Irvin D, Yu JS. Vaccination elicits correlated immune and clinical responses in glioblastoma multiforme patients. *Cancer Res*. 2008 Jul 15;68(14):5955-64.

[54] Wansley EK, Chakraborty M, Hance KW, Bernstein MB, Boehm AL, Guo Z, Quick D, Franzusoff A, Greiner JW, Schlom J, Hodge JW. Vaccination with a recombinant Saccharomyces cerevisiae expressing a tumor antigen breaks immune tolerance and elicits therapeutic antitumor responses. *Clin Cancer Res*. 2008 Jul 1;14(13):4316-25.

[55] Quenelle DC, Collins DJ, Rice TL, Prichard MN, Marciani DJ, Kern ER. Effect of an immune enhancer, GPI-0100, on vaccination with live attenuated herpes simplex virus (HSV) type 2 or glycoprotein D on genital HSV-2 infections of guinea pigs. *Antiviral Res*. 2008 Jun 23. [Epub ahead of print]

[56] Smahel M, Poláková I, Pokorná D, Ludvíková V, Dusková M, Vlasák J. Enhancement of T cell-mediated and humoral immunity of beta-glucuronidase-based DNA vaccines against HPV16 E7 oncoprotein. *Int J Oncol.* 2008 Jul;33(1):93-101.

[57] Park SH, Lee SR, Hyun BH, Kim BM, Sung YC. Codelivery of PEG-IFN-alpha inhibits HCV DNA vaccine-induced T cell responses but not humoral responses in African green monkeys. *Vaccine.* 2008 Jul 29;26(32):3978-83.

[58] Mehendale S, van Lunzen J, Clumeck N, Rockstroh J, Vets E, Johnson PR, Anklesaria P, Barin B, Boaz M, Kochhar S, Lehrman J, Schmidt C, Peeters M, Schwarze-Zander C, Kabamba K, Glaunsinger T, Sahay S, Thakar M, Paranjape R, Gilmour J, Excler JL, Fast P, Heald AE. A phase 1 study to evaluate the safety and immunogenicity of a recombinant HIV type 1 subtype C adeno-associated virus vaccine. *AIDS Res Hum Retroviruses.* 2008 Jun;24(6):873-80.

[59] Romero P. Current state of vaccine therapies in non-small-cell lung cancer. *Clin Lung Cancer.* 2008 Feb;9 Suppl 1:S28-36.

[60] Zhang C, Yu L, Qian R. Cloning and expression of Vibrio harveyi OmpK* and GAPDH* genes and their potential application as vaccines in large yellow croakers Pseudosciaena crocea. *J Aquat Anim Health.* 2008 Mar;20(1):1-11.

[61] Cipriani B, Fridman A, Bendtsen C, Dharmapuri S, Mennuni C, Pak I, Mesiti G, Forni G, Monaci P, Bagchi A, Ciliberto G, La Monica N, Scarselli E. Therapeutic vaccination halts disease progression in BALB-neuT mice: the amplitude of elicited immune response is predictive of vaccine efficacy. *Hum Gene Ther.* 2008 Jul;19(7):670-80.

[62] Waites KB, Canupp KC, Chen YY, DeVivo MJ, Nahm MH. Revaccination of adults with spinal cord injury using the 23-valent pneumococcal polysaccharide vaccine. *J Spinal Cord Med.* 2008;31(1):53-9.

[63] Rossi GR, Mautino MR, Awwad DZ, Husske K, Lejukole H, Koenigsfeld M, Ramsey WJ, Vahanian N, Link CJ. Allogeneic melanoma vaccine expressing alphaGal epitopes induces antitumor immunity to autologous antigens in mice without signs of toxicity. *J Immunother.* 2008 Jul-Aug;31(6):545-54.

[64] Amato RJ, Drury N, Naylor S, Jac J, Saxena S, Cao A, Hernandez-McClain J, Harrop R. Vaccination of prostate cancer patients with modified vaccinia ankara delivering the tumor antigen 5T4 (TroVax): a phase 2 trial. *J Immunother.* 2008 Jul-Aug;31(6):577-85.

[65] Redman BG, Chang AE, Whitfield J, Esper P, Jiang G, Braun T, Roessler B, Mulé JJ. Phase Ib trial assessing autologous, tumor-pulsed dendritic cells as a vaccine administered with or without IL-2 in patients with metastatic melanoma. *J Immunother.* 2008 Jul-Aug;31(6):591-8.

[66] Ge W, Li Y, Li ZS, Zhang SH, Sun YJ, Hu PZ, Wang XM, Huang Y, Si SY, Zhang XM, Sui YF. The antitumor immune responses induced by nanoemulsion-encapsulated MAGE1-HSP70/SEA complex protein vaccine following peroral administration route. *Cancer Immunol Immunother.* 2008 Jun 4. [Epub ahead of print]

Chapter XIII

CHAPERONE

WHAT IS CHAPERONE?

Terminology, chaperone means an adult who takes care of one or more unmarried men or women during social occasions. But this is not the medical specific meaning. In medicine, chaperone therapy is a new concept. Helping or assisting on other molecules is also the ways that chaperone acts. This term is primarily used in molecular biology. "How do chaperones operate in cells?" is a big scientific question [1]. Saibil said that recent advances were giving an improved understanding of the nature of chaperone interactions with their non-native substrate proteins [1].

Burston and Clarke said that chaperones could be broadly defined as proteins which interact with non-native states of other protein molecules and this activity was significant in the folding of newly synthesized polypeptides and the assembly of multisubunit structures; the maintenance of proteins in unfolded states fit for translocation across membranes; and the stabilization of inactive appearances of proteins which are switched on by cellular signals; and the stabilization of proteins unfolded during cellular stress [2]. Hartl said that different types of molecular chaperones, such as the members of the Hsp70 and Hsp60 families of heat-shock proteins, participate in a coordinated pathway of cellular protein folding [3-4].

Basically, Hsp70 proteins are central components of the cellular network of molecular chaperones and folding catalysts and these proteins could help a large variety of protein folding actions in the cell by transient relation to their substrate binding domain with short hydrophobic peptide segments within their substrate proteins [5-8]. Hsp90 is another molecular chaperone related to the folding of signal-transducing proteins, such as steroid hormone receptors and protein kinases [5-8]. Hsp90 contributes to several discrete subcomplexes, each having distinct groups of co-chaperones that function in folding pathways [5-8]. Wegele et al. said that the chaperones Hsp70 and Hsp90 might have a function in the folding and maturation of key regulatory proteins, like steroid hormone receptors, transcription factors, and kinases, some of which were related to cancer progression [7]. They noted that Hsp70 and Hsp90 construct a multichaperone complex, in which both are jointed by a third protein called Hop and such connection of and the interplay between the two chaperone machineries was of significant importance for cell viability [7].

Callebaut et al. noted that domain III, common to the hsp60s and hsp70s was also found in the hsp90s and adopts a beta-alpha-beta Rossmann-folded structure which was enrolled in the NAD-binding domain of dehydrogenases [8]. They noted that the hsp molecules could act as unfoldases by disrupting secondary structures through redox reactions on the main polypeptidic chain with which these molecules interact [8].

Table 1. Important reports on treatment using HSP70

Authors	Details
Jimbo et al. [12]	Jimbo et al. reported on induction of leukemia-specific antibodies by immunotherapy with leukemia-cell-derived HSP70 [12].
Chakraborty et al. [13]	Chakraborty et al. reported that resveratrol induces apoptosis in K562 (chronic myelogenous leukemia) cells by targeting a key survival protein, HSP70 [13].
Ren et al. [14]	Ren et al. reported on down-regulation of mammalian sterile 20-like kinase 1 by HSP70 mediated cisplatin resistance in prostate cancer cells [14].
Mizukami et al. [15]	Mizukami et al. said that both CD4+ and CD8+ T cell epitopes fused to heat shock cognate protein, HSP70 could function to eradicate tumors [15].
Zhou et al. [16]	Zhou et al. reported that dynamics and mechanism of HSP70 translocation was induced by photodynamic therapy treatment [16].
Bocci et al. [17]	Bocci et al. reported that ozonation of human blood could bring a remarkable upregulation of heme oxygenase-1 and HSP70 [17].
Kottke et al. [18]	Kottke et al. reported that induction of hsp70-mediated Th17 autoimmunity could be exploited as immunotherapy for metastatic prostate cancer [18].
Chang et al. [19]	Chang et al. reported on cancer immunotherapy using irradiated tumor cells secreting HSP70 [19]
Phillips et al. [20]	Phillips et al. reported on triptolide induces pancreatic cancer cell death via inhibition of HSP70 [20].

Chaperone Therapy

Chaperone therapy is a new concept of molecular therapy making use of chaperone. Modification of the folding is the action that brings therapeutic activity of chaperone. Guzhova said that since Hsp70 was found to disturb many signal pathways of apoptosis in many points, the high chaperone expression could lead to an increased resistance of tumor cells to anticancer drugs [9]. A 17-allylamino-17-demethoxygeldanamycin (17-AAG) is an anticancer agent currently in clinical trials [10]. This molecule represents a class of drugs, the benzoquinone ansamycin antibiotics, capable of binding and disrupting the function of Hsp90, leading to the depletion of multiple cancerous proteins [10]. Goetz et al. concluded that the Hsp90 chaperone complex was a novel target for cancer therapy [10]. Heike et al. noted that gp96, HSP70, and HSP90 are complexed to a diverse array of cellular proteins and peptides as a consequence of their chaperone functions [11]. Heike et al. said that these heat shock proteins complexes could be use in vaccines [11].

A. Treatment using HSP70

As previously mentioned, there are attempts to apply HSP70 in treatment. Important reports will be quoted and discussed in Table 1.

Table 2. Important reports on treatment using HSP90

Authors	Details
Sauvageot et al. [21]	Sauvageot et al. reported on efficacy of the HSP90 inhibitor 17-AAG in human glioma cell lines and tumorigenic glioma stem cells [21].
Shimamura et al. [22]	Shimamura et al. reported that Hsp90 inhibition could inhibit mutant EGFR-T790M signaling and overcomes kinase inhibitor resistance [22].
Hurtado-Lorenzo and Anand [23]	Hurtado-Lorenzo and Anand reported that HSP90 could modify LRRK2 stability and this finding implies potentials for Parkinson's disease treatment [23].
Holmes et al. [24]	Holmes et al. reported that silencing of HSP90 cochaperone AHA1 expression reduced client protein activation and expanded cellular sensitivity to the HSP90 inhibitor 17-allylamino-17-demethoxygeldanamycin [24].
Chatterjee et al. [25]	Chatterjee et al. reported that HSP90 inhibitors could attenuate LPS-induced endothelial hyperpermeability [25].
Sawai et al. [26]	Sawai et al. reported that inhibition of Hsp90 down-regulated mutant epidermal growth factor receptor (EGFR) expression and sensitized EGFR mutant tumors to paclitaxel [26].
Hemdan and Almazan [27]	Hemdan and Almazan reported that dopamine-induced toxicity was synergistically potentiated by simultaneous HSP-90 and Akt inhibition in oligodendrocyte progenitors [27].
Chandarlapaty et al. [28]	Chandarlapaty et al. reported that SNX2112, a synthetic HSP90, had potent antitumor activity against HER kinase-dependent cancers [28].

B. Treatment using HSP90

As previously mentioned, there are attempts to apply HSP90 in treatment. Important reports will be quoted and discussed in Table 2.

C. Treatment using gp96

As previously mentioned, there are attempts to apply gp96 in treatment. Important reports will be quoted and discussed in Table 3.

Table 3. Important reports on treatment using gp96

Authors	Details
Liu et al. [29]	Liu et al. reported on enhancement of cancer radiation therapy by use of adenovirus-mediated secretable glucose-regulated protein 94/gp96 expression [29].
Baker-LePain et al. [30]	Baker-LePain et al. said that glucose-regulated protein 94/glycoprotein 96 could elicit bystander activation of CD4+ T cell Th1 cytokine production in vivo [30].
Römisch [31]	Römisch reported that anti-bacterial defense relies on chaperone gp96 [31].

REFERENCES

[1] Saibil HR. Chaperone machines in action. *Curr Opin Struct Biol.* 2008 Feb;18(1):35-42.

[2] Burston SG, Clarke AR. Molecular chaperones: physical and mechanistic properties. *Essays Biochem.* 1995;29:125-36.

[3] Hartl FU. Principles of chaperone-mediated protein folding. Philos Trans R Soc Lond B *Biol Sci.* 1995 Apr 29;348(1323):107-12.

[4] Hartl FU, Martin J. Molecular chaperones in cellular protein folding. *Curr Opin Struct Biol.* 1995 Feb;5(1):92-102.

[5] Hartl FU, Martin J. Hsp70 chaperones: cellular functions and molecular mechanism. *Cell Mol Life Sci.* 2005 Mar;62(6):670-84.

[6] Bukau B, Horwich AL. The Hsp70 and Hsp60 chaperone machines. *Cell.* 1998 Feb 6;92(3):351-66

[7] Wegele H, Müller L, Buchner J. Hsp70 and Hsp90--a relay team for protein folding. *Rev Physiol Biochem Pharmacol.* 2004;151:1-44. Epub 2004 Jan 23.

[8] Caplan AJ. Hsp90's secrets unfold: new insights from structural and functional studies. *Trends Cell Biol.* 1999 Jul;9(7):262-8.

[9] Guzhova IV, Novoselov SS, Margulis BA. Hsp70 chaperone and the prospects of its application in anticancer therapy. *Tsitologiia.* 2005;47(3):187-99.

[10] Goetz MP, Toft DO, Ames MM, Erlichman C. The Hsp90 chaperone complex as a novel target for cancer therapy. *Ann Oncol.* 2003 Aug;14(8):1169-76.

[11] Heike M, Noll B, Meyer zum Büschenfelde KH. Heat shock protein-peptide complexes for use in vaccines. *J Leukoc Biol.* 1996 Aug;60(2):153-8.

[12] Jimbo J, Sato K, Hosoki T, Shindo M, Ikuta K, Torimoto Y, Kohgo Y. Induction of leukemia-specific antibodies by immunotherapy with leukemia-cell-derived heat shock protein 70. *Cancer Sci.* 2008 Jul;99(7):1427-34.

[13] Chakraborty PK, Mustafi SB, Ganguly S, Chatterjee M, Raha S. Resveratrol induces apoptosis in K562 (chronic myelogenous leukemia) cells by targeting a key survival protein, heat shock protein 70. *Cancer Sci.* 2008 Jun;99(6):1109-16.

[14] Ren A, Yan G, You B, Sun J. Down-regulation of mammalian sterile 20-like kinase 1 by heat shock protein 70 mediates cisplatin resistance in prostate cancer cells. *Cancer Res.* 2008 Apr 1;68(7):2266-74.

[15] Mizukami S, Kajiwara C, Ishikawa H, Katayama I, Yui K, Udono H. Both CD4+ and CD8+ T cell epitopes fused to heat shock cognate protein 70 (hsc70) can function to eradicate tumors. *Cancer Sci*. 2008 May;99(5):1008-15

[16] Zhou F, Xing D, Chen WR. Dynamics and mechanism of HSP70 translocation induced by photodynamic therapy treatment. *Cancer Lett*. 2008 Jun 8;264(1):135-44.

[17] Bocci V, Aldinucci C, Mosci F, Carraro F, Valacchi G. Ozonation of human blood induces a remarkable upregulation of heme oxygenase-1 and heat stress protein-70. *Mediators Inflamm*. 2007;2007:26785.

[18] Kottke T, Sanchez-Perez L, Diaz RM, Thompson J, Chong H, Harrington K, Calderwood SK, Pulido J, Georgopoulos N, Selby P, Melcher A, Vile R. Induction of hsp70-mediated Th17 autoimmunity can be exploited as immunotherapy for metastatic prostate cancer. *Cancer Res*. 2007 Dec 15;67(24):11970-9.

[19] Chang CL, Tsai YC, He L, Wu TC, Hung CF. Cancer immunotherapy using irradiated tumor cells secreting heat shock protein 70. *Cancer Res*. 2007 Oct 15;67(20):10047-57.

[20] Phillips PA, Dudeja V, McCarroll JA, Borja-Cacho D, Dawra RK, Grizzle WE, Vickers SM, Saluja AK. Triptolide induces pancreatic cancer cell death via inhibition of heat shock protein 70. *Cancer Res*. 2007 Oct 1;67(19):9407-16.

[21] Sauvageot CM, Weatherbee JL, Kesari S, Winters SE, Barnes J, Dellagatta J, Ramakrishna NR, Stiles CD, Kung AL, Kieran MW, Wen PY. Efficacy of the HSP90 inhibitor 17-AAG in human glioma cell lines and tumorigenic glioma stem cells. *Neuro Oncol*. 2008 Aug 5. [Epub ahead of print]

[22] Shimamura T, Li D, Ji H, Haringsma HJ, Liniker E, Borgman CL, Lowell AM, Minami Y, McNamara K, Perera SA, Zaghlul S, Thomas RK, Greulich H, Kobayashi S, Chirieac LR, Padera RF, Kubo S, Takahashi M, Tenen DG, Meyerson M, Wong KK, Shapiro GI. Hsp90 inhibition suppresses mutant EGFR-T790M signaling and overcomes kinase inhibitor resistance. *Cancer Res*. 2008 Jul 15;68(14):5827-38.

[23] Hurtado-Lorenzo A, Anand VS. Heat shock protein 90 modulates LRRK2 stability: potential implications for Parkinson's disease treatment. *J Neurosci*. 2008 Jul 2;28(27):6757-9.

[24] Holmes JL, Sharp SY, Hobbs S, Workman P. Silencing of HSP90 cochaperone AHA1 expression decreases client protein activation and increases cellular sensitivity to the HSP90 inhibitor 17-allylamino-17-demethoxygeldanamycin. *Cancer Res*. 2008 Feb 15;68(4):1188-97.

[25] Chatterjee A, Snead C, Yetik-Anacak G, Antonova G, Zeng J, Catravas JD. Heat shock protein 90 inhibitors attenuate LPS-induced endothelial hyperpermeability. *Am J Physiol Lung Cell Mol Physiol*. 2008 Apr;294(4):L755-8.

[26] Sawai A, Chandarlapaty S, Greulich H, Gonen M, Ye Q, Arteaga CL, Sellers W, Rosen N, Solit DB. Inhibition of Hsp90 down-regulates mutant epidermal growth factor receptor (EGFR) expression and sensitizes EGFR mutant tumors to paclitaxel. *Cancer Res*. 2008 Jan 15;68(2):589-96.

[27] Hemdan S, Almazan G. Dopamine-induced toxicity is synergistically potentiated by simultaneous HSP-90 and Akt inhibition in oligodendrocyte progenitors. *J Neurochem*. 2008 May;105(4):1223-34.

[28] Chandarlapaty S, Sawai A, Ye Q, Scott A, Silinski M, Huang K, Fadden P, Partdrige J, Hall S, Steed P, Norton L, Rosen N, Solit DB. SNX2112, a synthetic heat shock protein 90 inhibitor, has potent antitumor activity against HER kinase-dependent cancers. *Clin Cancer Res*. 2008 Jan 1;14(1):240-8.

[29] Liu S, Wang H, Yang Z, Kon T, Zhu J, Cao Y, Li F, Kirkpatrick J, Nicchitta CV, Li CY. Enhancement of cancer radiation therapy by use of adenovirus-mediated secretable glucose-regulated protein 94/gp96 expression. *Cancer Res*. 2005 Oct 15;65(20):9126-31.

[30] Baker-LePain JC, Sarzotti M, Nicchitta CV. Glucose-regulated protein 94/glycoprotein 96 elicits bystander activation of CD4+ T cell Th1 cytokine production in vivo. *J Immunol*. 2004 Apr 1;172(7):4195-203.

[31] Römisch K. Anti-bacterial defense relies on chaperone gp96. *Trends Biochem Sci*. 2001 Nov;26(11):644.

INDEX

A

B

C

D

F

G

I

J

K

N

O

P

T

U

V

W

X

Z